Migration and Intercultural Psychoanalysis

How does migration affect us in the deeper layers of our minds, where forces are at work that affect our mental and physical health, our experiences in the world and our behaviour?

This edited volume brings together contributions on the social, historical and personal aspects of migration from a psychoanalytic viewpoint. Clinical perspective is combined with a wider view that makes use of psychoanalytic concepts and experience to understand problematic issues around migration today. Later chapters take the historical background into account: the history of psychoanalysis itself is a history of migration, beginning with Freud's experiences of migration, in particular his flight from Vienna to London at the end of his life, to answer questions regarding migration, refugees, living in a 'multicultural society' and living in a 'foreign culture'.

Taking on the challenge of looking at the multi-layered, often subtle, yet powerful emotional and unconscious layers of meaning around migration, this book brings together practice and theory and will be of great interest to psychoanalysts, psychotherapists and those with an interest in the working of the mind in an intercultural context.

Kristin White is a psychoanalyst working with adults and children in her practice in Berlin, Germany. She is also a training analyst, lecturer and supervisor at the Alfred Adler training institute for psychoanalysis and psychotherapy in Berlin and a training member of the German Society for Psychoanalysis and Psychotherapy (DGPT).

Ina Klingenberg is a psychoanalyst and psychotherapist in Berlin, Germany. She took her psychoanalytic training in Berlin and Michigan and has a Masters in Psychoanalytic Cultural Science, Humboldt University. She has worked in cooperation with various organisations that provide support for refugees and migrants and is a trainee member of the German psychoanalytic associations DPG and DGPT.

Migration and Intercultural Psychoanalysis

Unconscious Forces and Clinical Issues

Edited by
Kristin White and Ina Klingenberg

Routledge
Taylor & Francis Group
LONDON AND NEW YORK

First published 2021
by Routledge
2 Park Square, Milton Park, Abingdon, Oxon OX14 4RN

and by Routledge
52 Vanderbilt Avenue, New York, NY 10017

Routledge is an imprint of the Taylor & Francis Group, an informa business

British Library Cataloguing-in-Publication Data
A catalogue record for this book is available from the British Library

Library of Congress Cataloging-in-Publication Data
A catalog record has been requested for this book

ISBN: 978-0-367-34238-8 (hbk)
ISBN: 978-0-367-63441-4 (pbk)
ISBN: 978-1-003-11922-7 (ebk)

Typeset in Times New Roman MT Pro
by KnowledgeWorks Global Ltd.

Contents

Contributors

M. Fakhry Davids is a psychoanalyst practising full-time in London. He is a Fellow and Training Analyst of the British Psychoanalytical Society, Honorary Senior Lecturer, Psychoanalysis Unit, University College London, and Visiting Lecturer, Tavistock Clinic, London. He is a Founding Board Member of Partners in Confronting Collective Atrocities (PCCA), and a Member of the EPF Ad Hoc Working Group on 'Psychoanalysis and Muslim Backgrounds'.

Cecilia Enriquez de Salamanca is a child and adolescent psychiatrist and psychoanalyst working in full-time practice with children and adolescents in Berlin. She is a member of the German Association of Child and Adolescent Psychiatry, Psychosomatics and Psychotherapy (BKJPP) and a lecturer and supervisor for infant and young child observation at the Institute for Analytic Child and Adolescent Psychotherapy ('IAKJP Esther Bick') in Berlin.

Nadja Gogolin is a psychoanalyst working in full-time practice in Berlin. She works with groups and with individuals and is a member of the German Psychoanalytic Society (DPG) and the German Society for Psychodynamic Group Psychotherapy (D3G). She is a member of the German Society for Psychoanalysis and Psychotherapy (DGPT) and a lecturer and group training analyst at three of the Berlin psychoanalytic and psychodynamic training institutes: BIPP, BAP und IfP.

Monika Huff-Müller is a psychoanalyst and a training analyst member of the German Society for psychoanalysis and Psychotherapy (DGPT) and the German Society of Adlerian Psychology (DGIP). She practises full-time in private practice in Aachen, Germany and is a training analyst and clinical supervisor at the Cologne Alfred Adler Institute for Psychoanalysis and Psychotherapy.

Ina Klingenberg is a psychoanalyst and psychotherapist practising full-time in Berlin, Germany. She works in cooperation with KommMit.e.V., an organisation that provides therapy for refugees. She is training to be a child and adolescent psychotherapist, is a trainee member of the German psychoanalytic associations DPG and DGPT and has a Masters in Psychoanalytic Cultural Science.

Ilany Kogan M.A. is a training analyst at the Israel Psychoanalytic Society. She is supervisor of the Psychotherapy Centre for Children and Adolescents in Bucharest. In addition, she works with groups on the topic of trauma and migration in Munich and Aachen, Germany. She previously worked as a clinical supervisor in Germany at the Department of Child and Adolescent Psychiatry in Eppendorf University Hospital and was also a member of the scientific advisory board of the Fritz Bauer Institute for Holocaust Studies in Frankfurt am Main, Germany. She was also a teacher and supervisor of the IPA Study Group in Istanbul, Turkey. In 2005, she received the Elise M. Hayman Award at the IPA congress in Rio de Janeiro for a study of the Holocaust and genocide. In 2016, she received the Sigourney Award for her lifetime work. She is the author of numerous books and journal articles, most notably her books, *The Cry of Mute Children, Escape from Selfhood* and *The Struggle Against Mourning.* A main focus of her work has been the study of the transmission of trauma from Holocaust survivors to the following generations as well as the treatment of the 'second generation' of Holocaust survivors, refugees and migrants.

Tülay Özbek is a psychoanalyst practising full-time in Berlin. She is a Fellow and Supervisor of the Karl Abraham Institute – Berlin Institute for Psychoanalysis (DPV) and founding member, lecturer and supervisor of the Berlin Seminar for Intercultural Psychotherapy and Supervision (BSIPS). A main focus of her work is the development of identity and self in the context of migration and globalisation and the specific problems and challenges for adolescents with hybrid cultural backgrounds.

Kristin White is a psychoanalyst in private practice, working with adults and children in Berlin, Germany. She is also a training analyst, lecturer and clinical supervisor at the Alfred Adler training institute for Psychoanalysis and Psychotherapy in Berlin and a training member of the German Society for Psychoanalysis and Psychotherapy (DGPT). She is also on the editing team of the German Adlerian psychoanalytic-psychotherapy journal *Zeitschrift für Individualpsychologie.*

Acknowledgements

This book is a selection of papers on the topic of psychoanalysis and migration that evolved out of the numerous discussions of a working group of psychoanalysts and psychotherapists in Berlin who work with English-speaking patients from all around the world. The working group is a self-organised further training group within the Berlin health administration (Kassenärztliche Vereinigung Berlin). We are thankful for the continuing support of the Berlin health administration, which has also helped to pay for some of the translations in this book. All the papers in this book and many others were read and discussed in great detail in the working group. Without the critical eye and the ongoing intellectual support of all the members of the working group, this book would not have come into being. As editors we would like to thank all the group members for their support, in particular, Deirdre Winter with her endless ideas for further reading, her lively interest in clinical methods and her specialist knowledge in the field of psychotherapy with traumatised refugees. Deirdre has also helped us with the translation or language issues of a number of the papers published here. We would also like particularly to thank Cecilia Enriquez de Salamanca from the same group, who has not only contributed with a paper from her specialised field of child psychoanalysis but also helped us with numerous content and editing suggestions.

We would also like to thank all our patients who have taught us so much about the conflicts and struggles, but also the joys of migration. Finally we would like to thank our senior production editor at Karnac, Nick Craggs and our copyeditor Pamela Bertram for their patience and all their helpful suggestions and corrections.

Introduction

Kristin White and Ina Klingenberg

This is a book for psychoanalytic practitioners working in the intercultural field or for those who are interested in the practice of psychoanalysis in an intercultural context.

One might think that there is nothing new about working as analysts with people from different countries and cultures or in languages that are not our own. Freud famously complained about his difficulties with the English language when he was offering psychoanalysis to the American patients who had become an essential source of income for him in the economic slump after the First World War:

> His linguistic failures, far less damaging than he imagined them to be, became something of an obsession. 'I listen and talk to Englishers 4–5 hours a day', he wrote to his nephew in July 1921, 'but I will never learn their d—d language correctly' … He found the '5, sometimes 6 and 7 hours' that he was listening to, and speaking in, English so 'strenuous,' he told Katja Levy late in 1920, that he could no longer answer letters at night and left that chore to Sundays.
>
> (Gay, 2006, pp. 388–9)

The face of migration has of course changed since Freud's day and is constantly changing as travel around the world becomes faster and more accessible to some of the world's population and available, but politically or financially inaccessible, to many others. In the face of these changes, intercultural psychoanalysis has become an issue. Questions are being asked, research conducted and psychoanalytic departments of intercultural psychiatry are being set up to meet the demand to understand and to help the many people seeking psychoanalysis in countries and languages that are not their own.

One basic and general question underlying all the chapters in this book concerns the effects of migration on the human mind. What are the factors that determine whether and how we are affected by experiences of migration? Each part of the book then addresses this question in relation to more specific aspects of intercultural psychoanalytic practice.

Part 1: Migration and defensive organisations

What are the various 'forces', internal as well as external, that lead to migration? Is migration always in some way traumatic? Are there specific themes, difficulties or pitfalls for the analyst working with people who have experienced migration? What about our analytic attitude in intercultural psychoanalysis? Can we ever be free of underlying prejudices towards 'foreigners' in our work as psychoanalysts?

Part 2: Languages, symbols and internal space

Can psychoanalysis be conducted in a language that is not the mother tongue of the patient or the analyst, or both? What is the effect of having different languages in the psychoanalytic situation? Do we as analysts have to know the culture, perhaps also the language from which our patients have come in order to conduct a psychoanalysis?

Part 3: Past generations, past worlds and the struggles of the patient in the present

What is the effect of migration through the generations? What is the effect of the many examples of migration in the history of psychoanalysis itself?

These are some of the issues that have been discussed over the years in our working group of English-speaking psychoanalysts and psychotherapists in Berlin, Germany. In Germany, around 300 hours of psychoanalytic psychotherapy are paid for within the state-aligned health insurance system. Thus, psychoanalysis or psychoanalytic psychotherapy is available for all those who need such treatment. Thus, the numerous cases discussed in this group over the years have not been wealthy patients migrating to Germany for their psychoanalysis and paying privately, like some of Freud's 'Entente people' (Gay 2006, p. 388), but patients from all walks of life in need of the help that psychoanalysis can provide.

The papers in this book have been chosen on the basis of many discussions in our working group and our many years of psychotherapeutic and psychoanalytic experience of working with English-speaking patients in Berlin. The papers address the above issues and questions in the light of psychoanalytic practice.

Reference

Gay, P. (2006). *Freud: A Life for Our Time*. New York, London: W.W. Norton & Co.

Migration and loss in a globalised world

Kristin White

'Home is where we start from' was the title of Winnicott's collection of essays (1986), quoting 'East Coker' from T.S. Eliot's *Four Quartets.* In the lines of poetry that follow, T.S. Eliot describes how, as we grow older, our experience of the world that began with the simplicity of 'Home' becomes stranger and more complex. Today, our world has grown and developed at a speed that we can hardly comprehend. The world has become 'global' and more complex. For many people, 'Home' is often no longer so easy to define.

We live in a world in which it has become an everyday phenomenon to fly across the globe, whether for work, holidays or to retain contact with friends and family. The ease with which migration takes place in the Western World and the fact that we now have a first-hand view of the world as a whole has brought with it both dangers and responsibilities. One of the psychic dangers is that we might lose ourselves in a narcissistic way, staying 'Up in the Air' (Reitman, 2009) in an internal 'conflict-free zone', losing touch with our internal home, without ever settling into a home.

But we also live in a world in which vast numbers of people are forced to migrate, to leave their home countries in search of a real, external 'conflict-free zone', a safe place to live and a place where their survival is not under threat. Modern media and fast travel around the world mean that we have immediate and direct knowledge of these groups of suffering fellow human beings who have been forced to migrate. These people may have lost their homes, seen their villages burnt down or had families killed in war zones. Here too, we can turn a blind eye to the truth and pretend that the suffering is not happening or that the people were never in any danger. We can try to deny any responsibility or experience any guilt as citizens of a globalised world. Sometimes borders are closed and walls and barbed-wire fences erected in an attempt keep an entire country in an illusory 'conflict-free zone'.

Addressing those conflicts, whether internal or external, is painful and often depressing, confronting us with uncomfortable truths, depressing realities and often helplessness. Yet this is the realm of psychoanalysis, an attempt not to look away but to confront painful truths in order to bring all the different and conflicting issues together in a much less perfect, but more integrated internal world. This book is a collection of papers in which psychoanalytic aspects of migration are addressed in different chapters.

The move away from one's home country, however liberating and however much desired it might be, will also involve painful feelings surrounding loss, which need to be addressed and understood. And each person's experience of loss will be personal and individual, depending on what has been left behind and what awaits him in the new country. As Freud remarked when he finally emigrated from Vienna, his home for so many years:

> The feeling of triumph on being liberated is too strongly mixed with sorrow, for in spite of everything I still greatly loved the prison from which I have been released. The enchantment of the new surroundings ... is blended with discontent caused by little peculiarities of the strange environment; the happy anticipations of a new life are dampened by the question: how long will a fatigued heart be able to accomplish any work?
>
> (Freud, 1938, p. 446)

Travel, emigration, learning new languages and discovering the world are of course not always related to neurosis, splitting or the avoidance of conflict. These processes can all be a trigger for new development and open the door to a playful and less rigid or narrow-minded view of reality.

Grinberg and Grinberg (1984) in their seminal work on psychoanalysis and migration, stress the importance of the early internalisation of good objects for a successful integration into the new culture. Internal hindrances that prevent the internalisation of good objects will make it more difficult for the individual to feel welcome in the new culture. The Grinbergs refer on numerous occasions to Winnicott and his theory of the 'intermediate area' or the 'potential space' where a child can develop a positive sense of being alone with himself in the presence of the good mother object. The positive sense of being alone with oneself without losing one's sense of identity is essential when a person is alone in a new culture. From a slightly different theoretical viewpoint, one might add the importance of the internalisation of a secure attachment relationship in which mentalising was able to develop, helping the individual to reflect on and understand his experiences in the new country. If on the other hand unconscious phantasies of a more attacking kind have developed in early childhood within an insecure or disorganised attachment relationship, then a more paranoid attitude to the new environment might develop after migration, making it much more difficult for a person to settle down or integrate into the new society.

One important aspect of psychoanalysis with migrants is that there can be no generalisations: each migrant is a person in his or her own right with her own personal history and her own personal struggles. This means that psychoanalytic treatment too, needs to be directed towards the personal, not generalised aspects of migration: '... In the case of multilingualism, every *technical* choice must derive from the specific relationship created in every single psychoanalytic situation' (Amati-Mehler, Argentieri and Canestri, 1993, p. 269).

Thus, this book is a collection of papers on the very personal and individual psychoanalytic struggles and joys with patients and analysts who have travelled, moved across the globe, learned and internalised various languages and have needed psychoanalytic understanding to integrate the migrant aspect of their internal selves.

References

Amati-Mehler, J., Argentieri, S., and Canestri, J. (1993). *Babel of the Unconscious: Mother Tongue and Foreign Languages in the Psychoanalytic Dimension*, trans. J. Whitelaw-Cucco. Madison, CT: International Universities Press.

Freud, S. (1938). Letter from Sigmund Freud to Max Eitingon, 6 June 1938. In Freud, E.L. (ed.) (1961) *Letters of Sigmund Freud 1873–1939*. London: The Hogarth Press pp. 444–6.

Gay, P. (1988). *Freud: A Life for our Time*. New York and London: W.W. Norton & Co.

Grinberg, R. and Grinberg, L. (1984). *Psychoanalytic Perspectives on Migration and Exile*. New Haven and London: Yale University Press.

Reitman, J. (dir.) (2009). *Up in the Air*, motion picture. Paramount Pictures, Los Angeles.

White, K. (2013). When migration is used as a defence against painful realities: Some experiences of working with English-speaking patients in Germany, *Psychoanalytic Psychotherapy*, *27*(1): 41–59.

Winnicott, D. W. (1986). *Home is Where We Start From: Essays by a Psychoanalyst*. New York and London: W.W. Norton & Co.

Migration in the first generations of psychoanalysts[1]

Ina Klingenberg

Seen historically, emigration has accompanied psychoanalysis from its beginnings. Freud himself had to immigrate as a young boy from Príbor (today the Czech Republic) to Vienna. Many of the early followers of Freud were also immigrants, such as Sándor Ferenczi and Sándor Radó. Often they came from Budapest. After the fascist Horhty Regime had taken over the government in Hungary (1920), they moved out of the country. At that time, the Budapest school was a very important psychoanalytic institution (Ferenczi was the first ever psychoanalytic university professor). Among these emigrants were Melanie Klein, Margaret Mahler, Alice Balint, Franz Alexander and more.

In the 1930s, emigration became an all-encompassing topic for psychoanalysts. It had so much influence on the development of the movement that some authors say that 'psychoanalysis was a history of migration' (Mühlleitner, 2005, p. 14), or they refer to the 'exodus of psychoanalysis'

(Handlbauer, 1999, p. 152). With the Nazi regime in power, first in Germany, then in Austria, almost all analysts had to migrate, some of them for the second or third time. In Berlin and Vienna – which were the main cities for psychoanalysis at that time – the psychoanalytic societies (German Psychoanalytic Society (DPG) and the Viennese Psychoanalytic Society (WPV)) were dissolved.

All Jewish psychoanalysts and politically active analysts were under immediate threat and sought refuge in countries outside the influence of the Nazi regime. Often they migrated several times, finding temporary homes in Paris, Prague, London or Zürich before finding their final destination, a place where they could settle permanently.

In Germany, the movement of migration, which had already started at the end of the 1920s, developed into the exodus of almost all psychoanalysts after 1933. In 1932, the German Psychoanalytic Society (DPG) had 56 members and 34 candidates. Roughly 100 psychoanalysts left the country, among them Melanie Klein, Karen Horney, Edith Jacobson, Hanns Sachs, Max Eitingon, Otto Fenichel, Wilhelm Reich, Theodor Reik, Georg Simmel and more.

In Austria, migration started more gradually in 1934, after the authoritarian Dollfuss Regime came to power. Helene Deutsch and Siegfried Bernfeld were among those who left the country even before the 'Anschluss' (the annexation of Austria by Germany in 1938). After 1938, almost all of the remaining analysts had to leave, among them Freud and his family. Between 1902 and 1938, the Viennese Psychoanalytic Association had 150 members, 95 of whom left the country in 1938/39. Altogether, there were roughly 150 psychoanalysts and candidates who had to escape from their country.

The influence of these migratory movements on psychoanalysis – personally and theoretically – are presumably much greater than we are often aware. On the one hand, there are the 'external aspects' of the influence of the migration: the development of the theory after migration, the changes of the practice and the influence of the migrants on the societies of the host countries. The influence of migrant psychoanalysts on medicine, psychology and the humanities as well as on the culture in the US is obviously enormous.

On the other hand there are the 'internal aspects' of the migration: the influence on the mind, the emotions, the way of experiencing the self and the world, the anxieties, the conscious and unconscious phantasies, etc., in other words, on the inner world of the migrant analysts themselves. Unfortunately, there are not many accounts of these experiences from the analysts. In the literature, one finds different explanations for this. One of the reasons might be that the experiences were so overwhelming that they had to be partly suppressed or they were only partly ready to be symbolised. As so often, it was Sigmund Freud himself who was the one to talk about his own difficult experiences. After his flight from Vienna to London he wrote:

'Everything seems to be unreal. We are neither here nor there' (Handlbauer, 1999, p. 156). Another quote can be found in the memories of Kohut:

> I lived two different lives and there seemed to be no bridge between them ... I can't find suitable words for describing clearly how I felt at home. My parents, even my grandparents, spoke Viennese ... I was in every sense a part of my surroundings. And yet there was this incomprehensible split.
>
> (cited in Handlbauer, 1999, p. 158)

Presumably, the impact on the inner world of the analyst was huge – much more than meets the eye. Analysts then, as well as today might well have tended to 'turn a blind eye' on the issue. Knowledge of the external circumstances – as horrific as they might be – does not necessarily reveal much about the way a particular afflicted person has experienced and processed those circumstances in his/her internal world. The same applies to our migrant patients now as it did to migrant analysts before.

This is highly relevant for our everyday psychoanalytic practice. One can assume that almost every analyst or trainee analyst has today at least one migrant psychoanalyst in his/her ancestry of training analysts. As psychoanalysts, we believe that during our training analysis, conscious and unconscious information and experiences are passed on from each training analyst to each candidate, from one generation to another. Words, atmosphere, emotions, associations etc. always transport unconscious, but meaningful material. From this point of view, it is very likely that in almost every training analysis, experiences of migration are somehow in the room – at least at some points during the analysis, even though the analyst and the trainee might not be aware of it. As analysts, we believe in the transport of meaningful but unconscious content through the generations. Presumably, these parts of our (training) experience will be mobilised – consciously or unconsciously – when we work with migrants. They might be a source of empathy for the patient, or they might evoke unconscious defences such as idealisation or lack of empathy for the migrant patient. In any case, we may presume that different levels of our own migration experience influence our everyday work with migrant patients in some way.

The third part of this book will deal with trans-generational aspects of psychoanalysis and with the history of the psychoanalytic movement. We hope to open up further discussion and thoughts about the connection between today's practice and the past experiences of the psychoanalytic movement with reference to migration.

'Migration and emigration are one of the big challenges of our day. We do not know if we are sufficiently prepared to face the conflicts that accompany it', said the German psychoanalyst C.E. Walker (DPV/IPA) at the beginning of a 2012 conference on Psychoanalysis and Migration in Berlin. Referring to the past, he continued 'For all of us it is a duty to remember [i.e. the history of Nazi Germany and the forced migration of psychoanalysts (I.K)] and to play our part in making sure that something like that does not repeat itself' (Hermann, Henningsen and Togay, 2013, p. 17).

Note

1. Translations by Ina Klingenberg

References

Handlbauer, B. (1999). Über den Einfluss der Emigration auf die Geschichte der Psychoanalyse [On the influence of migration on the history of psychoanalysis], *Forum der Psychoanalyse*, *15*, 151–66.

Hermann, M., Henningsen, F. and Togay, J.C. (eds). (2013). *Psychoanalyse und Emigration aus Budapest und Berlin* [Psychoanalysis and Emigration from Budapest and Berlin]. Frankfurt am Main: Brandes & Apsel.

Mühlleitner, E. (2005). Das Ende der Psychoanalytischen Bewegung in Wien und die Auflösung der WPV [The Ending of the Psychoanalytic Movement in Vienna and the Closure of the Viennese Psychoanalytic Association], in Wiener Psychoanalytische Vereinigung (ed.) *Trauma der Psychoanalyse* [Trauma of Psychoanalysis]. Vienna: Mille-tre Verlag.

Part I

Migration and defensive organisations

Part I of this book looks at specific themes, difficulties and pitfalls that analysts might experience in their work with people from different cultures and countries around the world.

John Steiner has written about 'psychic retreats' in which the internal reality of painful and frightening feelings and phantasies is avoided, often by 'turning a blind eye' to the truth, just as King Oedipus turned a blind eye when he gouged his eyes out, unable to face the unbearable truth that he had murdered his father and married his mother:

> Mechanisms such as 'turning a blind eye' which keep facts conveniently out of sight and allow someone to know and not to know simultaneously can be highly pathological and lead to distortions and misrepresentations of the truth ... Oedipus adopts a state of mind which can be thought of as a psychic retreat from reality and a defence against anxiety and guilt.
>
> (Steiner, 1993, p. 129)

The globalisation of our economy and our first-hand knowledge of social and political developments around the globe bring with it not only new horizons but also a new dimension of responsibility. As in the myth of Oedipus, many of us would like to gouge our eyes out and pretend not to see or take responsibility for the terrible plight of many of our fellow human beings who are trying to find safe havens in comparatively wealthy western societies. The political tendency to retreat into our small worlds, by closing the borders of our nations and trying to build up an illusion of privileged self-sufficiency in our economies and our food supplies, represents a socio-political version of a psychic retreat. When we recognise not only our dependency on the world as a whole and our responsibility towards the underprivileged, but also the role that hatred, envy, revenge and a drive towards superiority have played in the injustices of the world of which we are all a part, then our privileged position crumbles and we are left with a feeling of helplessness and humility in which as psychoanalysts we can merely do our best within our limited scope of effectiveness. Defences mounted against such feelings of helplessness and humility can lead to an attitude of intolerance of racial difference.

Both in the political sphere and on a personal level, the fear of loss and feelings of guilt and responsibility in the depressive position are in this way enacted instead of being worked through.

Reference

Steiner, J. (1993). *Psychic Retreats*. London: Routledge.

Chapter 1

Ethnic purity, otherness and anxiety: the model of internal racism[1]

M. Fakhry Davids

Introduction

Europe today has become increasingly multi-ethnic and multi-cultural. Borders between many of its nation states have come down, and inward migration from previously colonised developing world countries has added to a pleasing sense of diversity that, on the whole, continues to enrich the continent. Despite a degree of tension beneath the surface, it has by-and-large been possible to create a multi-cultural accommodation in which the values of tolerance and mutual respect prevail, often allowing individuals and communities to overcome states of enmity and hostility that, elsewhere, succeed in driving their ethnic, religious or cultural groupings apart. In Europe, however, people of many different shades and backgrounds have found a way to live reasonably comfortably side-by-side. If we consider the history of Europe in the 20th century, where the drive to set Jews and other minority groups apart from a supposedly truly native European essence – such as the model of Aryan purity – produced such devastating consequences, it does indeed appear that Europe has moved on. This can be seen, with some justification, as a major achievement.

Today, however, this accommodation is coming under strain from two sources. Firstly, there is the on-going threat of extremist violence, with groups such as al-Qaeda and Daesh determined to bring their on-going conflict with Western powers to the streets of Europe. The orchestrated attacks in Madrid on 11 March 2004, in London on 7 July 2005, in Paris on 13 November 2015, and in Brussels on 22 March 2016, are instances of this threat erupting into violent and deadly assaults on European citizens going about their day-to-day affairs. Such incidents set in motion psychic processes that tend to drive a wedge between Europeans of indigenous extraction and their Muslim and/or Arab compatriots.

A second source of tension stems from the unabated flow into Europe of refugees – fleeing war, instability, persecution, or poverty in their own African or Middle Eastern countries – desperate to make a new, safer and more secure home here. Germany, for example, faces the prospect of absorbing one million refugees from this influx in 2015 alone.[2] The pressure of integrating such very large numbers of new arrivals touches on primitive anxieties – for instance, will there be sufficient resources to go around? – that are readily articulated, especially by far-right groups, in racialised terms. The influx of refugees, particularly ones whose otherness is so visible, then comes to be seen as a threat to the very identity of western Europe as we know it. Is there a connection between this wish for a Europe, free of the 'other' in its picture of itself, and the Europe of yesteryear taken over by the pursuit of ethnic purity with such devastating consequences?

These are powerful social currents that draw all of us in, as citizens, bringing into the open, where they exist, racist mindsets that otherwise remain hidden. Even those with liberal attitudes can find their tolerance put to the test, and this may contribute to polarised thinking and political correctness, an atmosphere in which creative thought becomes more difficult. I have suggested that the model of internal racism can shed light on the psychological dimension of what is involved in these situations (Davids, 2002, 2006). In essence, I propose that there is a defensive system in the human mind, structured around the lines of racial/ethnic/cultural difference, which can be deployed in order to shield us from the profound anxiety generated in this situation. Stifling political correctness is one outcome of its deployment.

In addition to this broader perspective, internal racism is also directly relevant to psychoanalysts who may be called upon to treat patients from backgrounds distant from our own. Many refugees today come from a very different world, where they will have had deeply traumatic experiences, followed by an extremely stressful and perilous journey to Europe. These experiences need to be assimilated, and many may require professional help to do so and make an adjustment to their new homes. How well are psychoanalysts equipped to do this work? I want to suggest that an understanding of internal racism can assist us in preparing ourselves, internally, to do so.

The psychoanalytic study of racism

Racism is clearly a complex phenomenon. Sometimes it can be present with such devastating power that it sweeps away all sense and reason, almost effortlessly. Yet, at other times it can take the form of innocuous prejudice against an arbitrary out-group that can produce embarrassment, shame and guilt which, when faced, can genuinely move things forward.

It falls, of course, to psychoanalysis to give an account of how racism operates in the mind. This is more difficult than it seems. The psychoanalytic method proceeds best through clinical investigation, which one could do, for example, by revealing the inner workings of racism in a known racist. However, mostly even blatantly racist individuals deny their racism:

something other than racism is held responsible for beliefs and actions seen as racist by others. Moreover, when racists do seek help it is for difficulties other than their (disavowed) racism, and pursuing a full investigation into the nature of the racism in that patient's mind may pose an ethical dilemma in these cases: the analyst is in danger of prioritising his or her own research or theoretical interests above the patient's clinical concerns.

Cross-race analyses in general offer another way forward, and some have indeed been reported. An early classic was Wulf Sachs' *Black Hamlet*, in which Sachs, a Vienna-trained psychoanalyst working in Johannesburg, South Africa in the 1930s, tried to investigate psychodynamics in the mind of a black migrant worker (Sachs, 1937). It was not a conventional analysis – there was no therapeutic contract, meetings did not take place in a consulting room, etc. – and this was further complicated by the fact that Sachs clearly wanted to get something from the analysis in the way that an ordinary clinician would not. In fact, both introductions to the new edition of *Black Hamlet,* although sensitive to the fact that today's intellectual climate is very different from the one in which the study was undertaken, nonetheless draw attention to what would now be seen as implicitly racist attitudes that permeate it (Rose, 1996, Dubow, 1996). For instance, we can now recognise a hidden aim on the part of a white liberal working in a structurally racist society: to show that, beneath the skin, black and white were the same. Such hidden agendas restrict its scope for shedding light on manifestations of racism present in the rich and complex black–white transference that developed. For all its limitations, however, a contemporary re-reading of this work underscores two enduring points regarding the difficulty that psychoanalysis as a discipline has in engaging with the reality of racism. The first is that racism is an extremely slippery phenomenon that is hard to pin down in the consulting room. Donald Moss (2001) has suggested that racism is one of a class of phenomena for which it is very difficult to take personal responsibility – it is *we* who hate in racism, not *I* – and that this contributes to its slipperiness. A second enduring point is that an unconscious wish on the part of our profession to prove that human beings are, beneath the skin, made of the 'same stuff' (Thomas, 1992) may be implicated in our difficulty in engaging analytically with the reality of racism.

When psychoanalysts report on racist mechanisms at work in the minds of individual patients they tend to show how an individual patient uses a racial category, which helps to understand that patient's mind more fully (e.g. Schachter and Butts, 1968). However, extrapolating from this to a more general level, to the nature of racist mechanisms themselves, is problematic. Critics point out that psychoanalysts invariably seem to conclude that racism is a problem only because of underlying issues presumed to reside deeper within the psyche: racism is not the real issue. This, it is argued, is an *a priori* and hence untestable assumption; furthermore, this reductive turn is seen as defensive as it protects us from having to face the awkwardness of racialised encounters in the consulting room. This failure, in turn, partials out the very phenomena that should be the focus of any inquiry into racism, and so we remain unable to shed light on them. At worst, the resulting psychoanalytic discourse on racism becomes an unwitting instrument of the latter's perpetuation (Dalal, 2002).

The problem of reductionism to a psychological essence is serious and some of our colleagues, critical of the mainstream, think that as a discipline we just do not engage sufficiently with these issues. Instead, we are seen as smug and self-satisfied, which, it is argued, reflects a deeper bias within the psychoanalytic movement. Psychoanalysts, on the whole white, Western and privileged, are seen as best at analysing people like themselves (Perez Foster, 1996) since 'psychoanalytic assumptions on the nature of … psychological functioning are more loaded with Western cultural meanings than we commonly recognise' (Roland, 1996, p. 71). Patients who, in their outside lives, are the objects of racism find this very distressing. They feel that their actual experience as members of groups systematically discriminated against is denied; instead, they are perceived as someone else – beneath the skin really Western, middle class and white (Kareem, 1988). From this critical base, some progressive clinicians have moved away from traditional psychoanalysis and gone on to develop alternative models of therapeutic practice seen as more sensitive to the context of these 'other' groups (Kareem, 1992; Perez Foster, Moskowitz, and Javier, 1996; Roland, 1996).

I myself have taken a different approach that has led me to the formulation of a model of internal racism (Davids, 2011), which I shall outline briefly. I begin by asking, what are the elements of a racist object relationship that require psychological explanation? I examine a recognised racist interaction in the outside world to identify these elements, and turn to the consulting room to deepen the inquiry into them. I describe what I experienced, in my countertransference, as a racist attack launched on me in a session and, from knowledge of the patient gained over the course of a long analysis, I show how that attack stemmed from internal racism mechanisms mobilised in the patient's mind. I go on to suggest that these mechanisms belong to the normal mind – not his unique psychopathology – and give meaning to the aspects of racist interchanges identified earlier, as they occur both in the world and in the consulting room. I then discuss the relevance of this understanding to our changing world today.

Racism in the world

In the real world racism has a concrete existence, and always involves a perpetrator and victim – the racist subject and the object of his/her racism. How to designate them, however, is already difficult and thorny. To speak of the racist subject and the object of racism would be most correct, but academic and clumsy; to speak of perpetrator and victim calls forth undesirable associations – victimhood, for instance, carries negative and disempowering connotations.

One way forward is to begin with an obvious incarnation of racism, such as that on the part of the indigenous, white, empowered group against non-white, disadvantaged, immigrant groups and their descendants – white–black racism. Such an approach would be difficult to justify in a purely academic paper, where one would be expected to begin with a more precise definition of the term racism. However, in a psychoanalytic inquiry this is a good enough starting point from which to explore whether a deepening of our understanding of racism is possible. The terms 'black' and 'white' themselves are nevertheless problematic. As far as description is concerned, the natives' skin colour is never literally white – it ranges from pinkish-grey to light yellow-brown – and non-white has the disadvantage of designating real, live persons negatively – as 'not something'. Put another way, these ways of designating subject and object involved in a racist interaction are already racialised (Dalal, 2002). Psychoanalytically, this is to recognise that the terms we usually employ involve an empty racial category (Rustin, 1991) being saturated with psychic content: something has been done to brown pale and skin to turn them black and white respectively. This something is part of what needs to be understood. My use of these terms is therefore schematic.

Let me begin with a description of an actual racist attack on the streets of London (Macpherson, 1999). Late one night in April 1993, a group of racist thugs killed a black teenager, Stephen Lawrence, who was waiting for a bus with a friend. A lack of credible evidence meant that no one was tried for his murder. For many this situation was seen as an example of the indifference of officialdom, which enshrines the principle of equality for all its citizens, yet seems oblivious to the existence of anti-black racism. In response to complaints of institutionalised racism, an internal police inquiry exonerated the police of all blame, a conclusion endorsed by the Conservative government of the day. It was only in the wake of the latter's defeat in the general election of 1997 that a public inquiry into the police handling of the case was set up.

At the inquiry Duwayne Brooks described how, on the night in question, he and his best friend, Stephen, had been waiting for a bus in Eltham, south-east London, when six white youths approached. One of the youths yelled out, 'what, what, a nigger', and pulled out a large steel or wooden weapon with which he struck Stephen. Stephen screamed in pain and fell, but Duwayne helped him up and they started to run. However, Stephen faltered, saying he could not carry on, and when Duwayne looked back he saw his friend slumped to the ground, blood on his jacket. Duwayne rushed to phone for an ambulance and tried to stop passing cars, all the while frightened that it was too late – 'I saw his life fading away'. When the police arrived, however, they seemed to be repulsed by the blood and ignored Duwayne's pleas for them to drive Stephen to a nearby hospital. And when he pointed out to the police the road where their assailants had fled, the policewoman 'did nothing'.

Away from the heat of the incident, it seems to us that any reasonable person coming upon such a scene would have two priorities in mind: first to get help to the wounded boy, and then to pursue any lead that might allow those responsible to be apprehended. If we accept, as the inquiry was told, that PC Bethel – the policewoman involved – was an ordinary, conscientious police officer, then something happened at the scene to seriously interfere with her capacity to function in her ordinarily good and conscientious way. She probably felt that, by keeping in mind that Duwayne Brooks might just be his friend's assailant, she was merely doing her duty. He, however, on the receiving end, experienced it differently:

> 'It was like she didn't believe me ... she was treating me as if she was suspicious *of me*, not like she wanted to help,' he said ... 'I am sad and confused about this system where racists attack and go free, but innocent victims like Steve and I are treated like criminals.'
>
> (*The Guardian*, 16 May 1998, italics added)

Duwayne Brooks felt that the police officer viewed him in a racist way, a point pursued at length in the inquiry. The assertion is that something racist in her was responsible for her momentary loss of perspective; had this not happened, she would have functioned in her usual way and got her priorities right.

The possibility that Stephen might be bleeding to death, or that other possible suspects were making good their getaway, would have been paramount in her mind. I want to pursue that same point, but in a more specific way, by suggesting that the paralysis of one's ordinary professional functioning is linked with internal racism mobilised in the cross-race[3] encounter. This is my first observation, which I hope to investigate further.

On the morning after the murder, the police officer had recovered somewhat and felt burdened by guilt.[4] At that point the situation might have been rescued: although Stephen could not be brought back to life, everything might yet have been thrown into bringing his killers to justice, an act of reparation that might have mitigated that guilt. Instead, it seems that the possibility that something racist may have happened at the murder scene could not be faced, and the subsequent investigation was fatally undermined by further, quite extraordinary, police failures. Psychoanalytically, this suggests that the guilt was unbearable, and dealt with through re-enactment of the original failure. In retrospect, it is as if everyone, not just the police officer herself, felt unconsciously accused of racism and determined to protect themselves by closing ranks. As I indicated at the outset, this cover-up stretched to the highest levels. This is the second issue to be understood:

why is it that when racism is present we all seem so easily sucked in, and find it so hard to recover?

Internal racism

I will now describe a clinical encounter that alerted me to the existence of internal racist mechanisms, and allowed me to study its operation in some detail. Mr A[5] was an intelligent man who had an unremarkable childhood. Privately educated and always top of his class, he went on to boarding school, and then to university where, towards the end of his time, he began to struggle. After graduation he more or less broke down in his first job and never quite recovered. For some years he struggled on valiantly before realising that he needed help, but he came for psychoanalytic psychotherapy very reluctantly, having previously obtained limited help from less intensive forms of treatment – counselling, group psychotherapy, CBT etc. He ended up having a long, full analysis with me, and my understanding of the interchange I shall describe is informed by knowledge of his mind gleaned over many years.

Like his childhood, his first two sessions with me were also rather unremarkable. He described his background and the nature of his difficulties, but so intellectually that it was difficult to establish any emotional contact with him. Then, in his third session, he related the following incident: He had just learnt that his father would be furious with him over something he had done that clearly went against his father's wishes. While driving along in their new car he heard a strange noise coming from the engine, and became convinced that the car was about to explode. Fearing for his life, he stopped, got out and locked the door behind him, dropped the keys down a drain, and made for home. He then became terrified that his mother had committed suicide. He rang, and was immensely relieved when it was she who answered the phone.

Here he broke off, waiting for my response. I was thinking that the new car stood for the new therapy which he feared would blow up were he to be true to himself and risk a confrontation, rather than being the good, co-operative boy of the first two sessions. However, I realised that were I to put this to him, he would almost certainly respond to it intellectually, as before. Instead, I decided to focus my interpretation on the quality of his reaction to the strange sounds that came from the engine, i.e. that he was alerting me to something *within him,* so violent that it could not be tolerated, and thus had to be split off and projected into the engine, which, in turn, was not going to contain it.[6] As a first step, I said that he was telling me of an enormous rage within him, which, were it touched in his therapy, he feared I would not be able to cope with.

He was silent for a while, apparently mulling over what I had said. Eventually he replied in a reasonable but rather strained voice that it was always the same, his rage was always *so enormous*. Rage now took him over, rapidly growing out of control, and it became clear that he took my using the word *enormous* to be a complaint at the extent of rage that I saw in him. He became more and more furious, yelling abuse and accusations at me, all revolving around his perception that, by mentioning it so directly, I wanted him to suppress that rage and be 'good'. That way he would earn my approval and praise, which would somehow cure him. Yet this was the story of his life that had, in fact, led him to grief. Under no circumstances would he be fooled into following such a path again – why should it work this time?

During the very occasional lull in this onslaught, I tried to reach him through interpretation. For instance, I pointed out how he seemed to take my remark as a complaint. Or, that he was convinced I would not tolerate his rage but instead try to reason him out of it. However, such interventions did not reach him; they simply added fuel to the fire and he laid into me with renewed gusto.

When he left I was reeling from the sheer ferocity of his attack. At first I felt completely numb, then I found my mind scurrying down one alley after another, desperately seeking an explanation for the sudden switch in him. Gradually, I realised that this was an intellectual exercise designed to help me regain my emotional balance, and this helped me to appreciate how much I had been destabilised by the encounter. However, I found that I was unable to put a name to my feelings of extreme disturbance and discomfort, and following this realisation it became possible to put the matter aside and settle down to the rest of the day's work.

On my way home that evening a police car sped by, siren blaring and blue lights flashing. In my mind's eye I could see them stop and harass some hapless black man, just as I myself had been some years before. Feelings of being racially violated, of feeling immobilised and gripped by a helpless fury, came flooding back. Sometime later I realised that these feelings were identical to what I felt after Mr A's session, but could not name; I had felt *racially* attacked. This puzzled me, as my patient was not a racist. On detailed reflection I could find no hints of anything racist in his material and concluded that my own hypersensitivity to such matters made me sense a racial attack where, in fact, there had been none. I thus put it out of my mind.

In the following session, however, I reconsidered this when Mr A discussed at some length his fear that, on account of my being a foreigner, I would not be able to understand him fully. This confirmed that he had been aware of the difference between us – he was a native Englishman, I am brown-skinned and obviously foreign (perhaps of Middle Eastern or near Asian extraction) – and I could now consider my feeling racially attacked as a countertransference response.

My patient was very ill – he went on to have a psychotic breakdown in the course of the analysis – with a damaged internal object[7] felt to be completely incapable of psychological 'holding'. Because of the absence in his mind of someone who could contain his infantile anxieties – all of which were mobilised by the act of seeking help – he could not imagine that anything good might come from his impending involvement with me. Yet he also realised that he had no choice. This was an impossible dilemma, which I think he resolved in the following way: in the moment that he laid eyes on this foreigner, an *internal racist organisation* opportunistically took shape in his mind. At the core of that organisation stood a me into whom his needy infantile self had been projected.[8] Following this projection it was I, not he, who faced a desperate struggle to survive in a hostile world whilst he was freed to be the co-operative gentleman of the previous two sessions.

That initial projective identification was based on an accurate perception of me as brown-skinned and foreign. But this perception was most fleeting, as, in the next moment it gave way, imperceptibly, to a second perception, that of me weighed down by a daily struggle against widespread forces of institutional racism. Now, in his eyes, I was a black man to whom whites did terrible things. Projective identification across the colour divide had taken place, and he himself was no longer burdened by conflicts over dependency: I met a gentleman. Moreover, his perception of me now allowed him to evade responsibility for my plight. He was not racist or xenophobic and felt that the forces of institutional racism in society were a cancer that should be rooted out. *He* would want me to be at home here; the British National Party[9] would not. Note that these considerations are underpinned by an assumption that it is I who faced the problem of whether the world I find myself in could ever really be my home, and this would have reassured Mr A that his projection of the infant riddled with dependency problems was successful. The man he saw in front of him really did have that struggle.

When I speak of a racist *organisation* in the patient's mind it is to draw attention to the fact that once the processes I have just described (projective identification across an external divide) are in place, further work was done to construct an inner template that was to govern relations between us. Once in place, the demand was that we should both play our roles allotted by the organisation. His was to be 'co-operative'; mine was to listen sympathetically and to discuss with him his past and outside problems with a view to understanding them intellectually (like two gentlemen), but I was not to touch him emotionally. This arrangement kept at bay any awareness that he needed me in an ordinary way, as any patient does their therapist. I think I sparked off his vicious attack by stepping out of line when I made an interpretation in the transference regarding a fear that I would not be able to contain his rage. This of course implied that he *needed* me to do so. For the most fleeting of moments this interpretation touched him, bringing a glimmer of awareness of dependency. However, this was the very thing that the racist organisation was designed to rescue him from. What followed was, therefore, a desperate attempt to turn my interpretation into a complaint:

if I complained I *wanted* something else from him. We would then be in our proper roles in relation to each other, and the fleeting awareness of need in him would have been reversed. Note that this attack was directed not at my foreignness or blackness but at my functioning as an ordinary psychotherapist. The attack was racist in that it was designed to force me back into my allocated 'black' role.

Racist and pathological organisations

My understanding of the internal racist organisation is derived from John Steiner's concept of the pathological organisation. Steiner (1987, 1993) argues that the pathological organisation functions as a refuge from primitive emotional states: the terrors of the paranoid-schizoid position on the one hand, and the unbearable pain of the depressive position on the other. The individual feels safely protected from these internal situations as long as he lives psychically within the pathological organisation, which is believed to afford mafia-like protection in return for mafia-like loyalty. This means that all interactions with the object must be seen to conform to the parameters of the organisation. I think the internal racist organisation serves the same purpose, and functions in the same way as a pathological organisation.

An internal racist organisation shifts the psychic focus towards ensuring that interactions conform to a structured inner template – that everyone keep to their proper place. This helps to keep out of awareness the fact that an arbitrary attribute of a person (e.g. skin colour) was chosen to justify massive projection into them, which is of course recognisably racist. My patient had no pause for thought – he just found himself faced with a black man who faced terrible problems on the street, which he, thankfully, did not; by then both my brown and his pale skin had been racialised through projective identification. Usually the only conscious derivative of this process is the attempt to justify one's view of the object by proving that the perceptions on which they are based are actually true (blacks *do* smell; Jews *do* control the world; Muslims *are* intolerant fanatics). My patient did so when he insisted that, burdened as I was by my black skin, I wanted him to be no trouble; this he knew for sure.

Once relationships are organised in accordance with such stereotypes, the object of internal racism is recruited, willy-nilly, to play out a role in someone else's 'inner dream script', the setting up of which can be thought of as analogous to Freud's description of the dream work (Freud, 1900). This is an invasive process with power to eat away at the object's sense of him-/herself as a person, part of which derives from the fact that it is played out unconsciously. However, while the subject may be unaware of it the object, at the receiving end, usually feels its impact fully: he *is not and must not be* an ordinary person.[10] Thus, the police officer could, in all innocence, feel that she was just doing her job while Duwayne Brooks *felt* something racist happening; Mr A was just objecting to my unreasonable 'complaint' about him but I *felt* racially attacked. These experiences appear as if out of the blue: in fact, they happen at the precise moment when the 'what, what, a nigger?' role is thrust upon the object with such force that there is no escape.

I have been describing ways in which the internal racist organisation is like the pathological organisation. There are, however, two crucial differences between the two. First, whereas a pathological organisation results from something going wrong in the course of development, the internal racist organisation is an outcome of development that has proceeded normally. It develops to help the child bind primitive anxiety, at a stage when it is already sufficiently attuned to external reality to have an awareness of real social stereotypes. These are given a new, individually charged, lease of life as they are assimilated to become an integral part of the beliefs about the 'racial' other. I have outlined its developmental trajectory elsewhere (Davids, 2011). Second, although these are beliefs about the other are held to be true, the fact that they belong to a phantasy system remains concealed; the individual concerned believes they reflect external reality as it is. Thus, for example, the immigrant is seen as so desperately needy that he threatens our livelihood. Because these stereotyped beliefs are accepted as true within one's social milieu, the fact that they belong to a phantasy construction remains hidden. This gives it extraordinary power.

Ordinarily, our internal racism does not cause problems, as its contents remain private and hence contained; they do not interfere with our ability to adapt to reality. An out-group is, after all, outside the range of our ordinary experience, hence members of that group are ideally placed to become containers for racist projection. However, there is a price to pay for our internal racism: in our professional encounter with someone from a different cultural/ethnic background we enter onto pathological organisation terrain in the mind, mobilising anxieties so intense as to de-skill us and paralyse our ordinary functioning. This is what I think happened to the police constable, and it happened to me when I felt numbed after my patient left. It is an observation that can be made repeatedly, and indicates, I think, that each and every one of us has an internal racist tucked away in a corner of our mind. In addition, when we get tangled up with something racist within, these same mechanisms are triggered in those around us, making it hard for them to be of real help.

Living with our internal racism

By emphasising that we all have internal racism in us I hope to shift the focus from *whether* to *how* we are racist, and this is important for the psychoanalyst for two reasons. Firstly, as I have already indicated, many members of minority ethnic groups complain that analysts do not properly attend to their experience of racism. To do so requires a conceptual grasp of racism in the mind. Secondly, while internal racism might not, under ordinary circumstances, pose a problem it is readily mobilised in the cross-race/cultural setting, where it can turn matters racial into a no-go area (e.g. Hamer, 2002). If this paralysis in the consulting room is to be overcome, it is essential for the clinicians first to face their own internal racism. Yet this may require more tolerance of our racism than our liberal instincts permit. What follows is a schematic picture of the terrain on which internal racism is located, and therefore of the sorts of issues that need to be faced.

The first issue is to locate the object of our internal racism. For some this will be members of a particular racial group, for others language/religious groups; some are familiar with the objects of their racism (i.e. they can own their racism), while others parade a pseudo-tolerance that carries no emotional resonance ('some of my best friends are Jews'). Yet others project the racist within into someone else (e.g. a parent who wants their daughter to marry within the family/clan/faith etc), leaving them apparently free but immobilised, through projective identification, by the object's prejudices, and powerless in the face of it.

Whether owned or projected, internal racism is underpinned by a belief about the object that is held with absolute conviction – external evidence will usually be adduced to support it – and this justifies the particular, fixed mode of relating to him or her. This makes racism invasive: it leaves no room for the object to be an ordinary human being; s/he is co-opted into being the object of racism.

Reaching an accommodation with the internal racist requires, as a first step, that we locate its emotional heart and that we enter that area. This can be extremely difficult to do since racist organisations do not simply roll over and give up once the light of awareness shines upon them. On the contrary, they are extremely resilient structures capable of numerous new permutations that preserve intact their fundamental structure whilst yet possibly conceding one or two matters of detail. This is the fundamental problem that blacks will refer to as 'tokenism': a token black is recruited in order to give the appearance of a non-racist institution, and this in itself is the means to resist true scrutiny that might lead to real change.

Once we gain access to the area of the mind where internal racism is located, we are on sensitive mental terrain in which a characteristic nexus holds sway, comprised of intense emotion, primitive defences, and unbearable pain and guilt, accompanied by a paralysis of what Freud called secondary process functioning (including the capacity to think). This is because the internal racist organisation, like the pathological organisation, is a refuge from both paranoid-schizoid and depressive anxieties. Any movement beyond its confines immediately exposes us to these primitive anxiety situations, which will be familiar to all who have tried to grapple with cross-cultural/racial issues.

On the paranoid end, one is *accused* of being a racist, and is damned; anything said in one's defence makes it worse; the only thing to do is to own up and atone; or one is a virtuous victim of racism, thus both saved and saviour. One becomes the authority on racism and all that is associated with it. The atmosphere easily turns hostile and suspicious, it is not possible to think, and political correctness becomes the order of the day. We feel divided into friends and enemies.

At the depressive end, to own one's racism brings guilt, which is felt to be so heavy that it cannot be borne. Think of that poor police officer having to live with the thought that, had she listened to Duwayne Brooks and rushed Stephen Lawrence to hospital, he might be alive today. Or, had she followed his lead, the killers might be behind bars instead of triumphantly walking the streets, to strike again who knows when? Or think of a white woman who, in a race awareness group, insisted that they, the white people of the world, had to accept responsibility for the sins of colonialism, since the white world still reaps its benefits. The weight of guilt was palpable; of course, projecting into someone *is* a form of colonial occupation. Or think of the acceptance by the Commissioner of the London Metropolitan Police that racism may be inherent in his force, only vehemently to deny charges of institutional racism. As he sees it, this would mean that all members of his force, whom he knows to be basically good people, wilfully intend to commit racist acts in the course of carrying out their duty. This gives voice to an anxiety that when responsibility for racism is truly accepted, the fear is of guilt so overwhelming that it would be unbearable; it would wash away almost any redeeming qualities one might have.

Clinical application

These issues are painful and distressing, but they do need to be faced if we are to function optimally as clinicians in the cross-race/culture encounter. Let me give an example that comes from Europe in another era that will demonstrate what I mean.

Jafar Kareem (1988) describes how profoundly disturbing an experience the encounter between a patient from a developing world background and a native European clinician can be. Kareem, a young clinical psychologist of Indian descent based in England, had travelled to Vienna to work and gain experience in psychoanalysis. He became depressed and consulted a woman psychoanalyst.

In the fifth session he recounts a short dream: 'It is during the uprising against the British in India. He is on a march with his fellow students when they are confronted by a mass of policemen with red turbans. Suddenly, shots erupt and the friend next to him is shot and lies bleeding on the ground. Meanwhile, the police drag Kareem away to a waiting black van'. He associates the red turbans with the analyst's red scarf.

At first the analyst reprimands him for going on a march – 'Didn't your parents tell you not to take part in such things?'. Eventually she interprets that the British authorities, whom he and his friends are rebelling against, stand for the father he had lost within a month of his birth. Kareem protests that though, indeed, he had no memory at all of his father, a number of uncles seemed to have been good enough surrogate fathers to him. He goes on to insist on a transference link: in the dream the analyst was 'behind the police' in a vague sort of way – a reference to his associating their red turbans with her red scarf. She now interprets that he holds all Europeans responsible for his oppression, in a way that underlines the irrationality of such a view ('Maybe you think we all shot your friend'), and suggests that he wishes to take revenge on her for this (Kareem, 1988, pp. 58–62). Following that session Kareem terminates the treatment.

How can we understand what went wrong? The analyst's working hypothesis is a reasonable one that has two components: first, that the dream records his protest against an authority felt to be not only unjust but also tyrannical and murderous in stifling the protest itself; and second, the protest concerns parental failure – identified as the absence of a proper father – stirred up by the analyst in the transference. One might say this is a standard psychoanalytic formulation, which takes no account of the difference in cultural/ethnic background between analyst and patient and its meaning in the here-and-now. As I mentioned earlier, intercultural critics of psychoanalysis would maintain that this reflects its hidden prejudice against patients from non-Western backgrounds. The model of internal racism outlined above, on the other hand, would suggest that these mechanisms contributed to the breakdown of this treatment in a specific way.

The analyst's interpretation of the dream is based on the understanding that Kareem's depression connects with unconscious aggression against an unavailable object, a proposition for which there is theoretical and clinical support (Freud, 1917). However, I think this idea is used to defend the analyst from even greater anxieties related to their ethnic/cultural difference that is alive between them in the here-and-now.

In the initial interview, despite the fact that Kareem was a psychologist who had travelled to Vienna in part to gain experience of psychoanalysis, the analyst explicitly called into question whether he was aware that psychotherapy is a sophisticated undertaking based on complex psychoanalytic theory, and was lengthy and costly. At the end of the interview, she checked whether he knew how to use a telephone (in case he should need to ring her) since 'the telephone is a western thing'.

Today, some 40–50 years after the event, we could easily recognise that the analyst was racially stereotyping her Indian patient and, in the process, reducing a depressed younger colleague to a miserable, backward and uncivilised foreigner. The patient clearly experienced this racist assault acutely, and we could see the aggression in the dream as directed not towards an unavailable object (the father he lost) but towards one who failed him – rather than see him as he is she saw him through a racially stereotyped lens. I think the anxiety alive at that moment, articulated by the dream, involved his experience of her as a European racist. I would like to pause here to discuss this in more detail.

In today's Europe there are many more brown-skinned individuals – visible members of recent immigrant groups – than during Kareem's time. Thus, while the encounter with a minority-group patient may still be a novel experience for the analyst, today this would not be the alien one that it clearly was for the first analyst. How might this influence the dynamic between them? I think we are all now much more aware that remarks such as hers give offence as they either are, or are felt to be, racist, and thus they go against our liberal instincts. We would thus avoid them. But does this stance reflect political correctness rather a resolution of the racist response at a deeper level? Here the feeling of the analyst holds the key. The model of internal racism suggests that if the analyst feels immobilised emotionally, paralysed, like the police constable at the murder scene I described earlier, this indicates that internal racist mechanisms are alive within the analyst. It is then imperative, in my view that the analyst attends to this inner situation.

Let me return to Kareem's account to take our discussion forward. After breaking off with the first analyst he proceeded to a second, to whom he related the same dream. That analyst put into words Kareem's hatred of European oppressors (based on the association between the red of the first analyst's scarf and the police turbans in the dream), saying that it is something whose full meaning is, at the beginning of the treatment, yet unknown. He went on to add that his patient was now in Austria, which had a history of collaboration with the Nazis. Whose side had he, the analyst, been on? This acknowledges that the problem was not confined to India, as in the dream. In Europe, too, a regime was in place built on the idea of the superiority of the putatively native Europeans, the Aryans, which murderously targeted Jews whose oriental origin was seen as polluting the landscape. In addition, he acknowledges explicitly that the question of where the analyst stood in this was relevant between them. Was he too, 'behind the police in some kind of way'? It is only after all of this is verbalised that he goes on to acknowledge that a great deal is as yet unknown about these matters, both between them and in the patient's mind; and to raise the question of whether they could work together to explore it. This strikes a completely different note to the first clinician and it comes as no surprise that this second treatment proceeded to a satisfactory outcome.

It is clear, then, that though the first clinician was very involved in the racial dynamic between them, she remained blind to this fact. I think it is this blindness that gives her interventions a ham-fisted and clumsy feel, even though they were derived from a plausible psychoanalytic hypothesis. Note, in passing, that the second analyst uses this same formulation (that depression involves aggression against the object) but translates it into quite different interventions, recognising that in the dream aggression is directed, in the first instance, at the European oppressor, and finds in this an opportunity for locating it directly between them. Faced with her patient's doubts regarding her interpretation the first analyst, on the other hand, becomes more and more defensive and her interventions lack the creativity and nimbleness of mind we all strive for as clinicians. We might also note that her chosen line of interpretation moves directly to the patient's past unconscious, and in the process bypasses completely unconscious dynamics alive in the present (Sandler and Sandler, 1987).

I want to suggest that one factor that may have contributed to this state of affairs is the absence of a coherent model of how racist dynamics work in the mind (Leary, 2000). This deprives the clinician of a tool necessary to conceptualise that aspect of the cross-race/culture clinical encounter, which in turn limits his or her ability to process the experience properly. The model of internal racism described in this paper is an attempt to meet this need.

I am aware that I have written the above account based on the narrative of a patient rather than an analyst. This does not imply that I accept Kareem's account of the interchanges between himself and his first analyst as true. However, it is his account, and if it were not true then the racism he attributes to his analyst would be seen as emanating from his own mind: his racialised hatred of the European other is projected into the analyst. Even if this were the case, it would nonetheless be the analyst's responsibility to address it, which she clearly could not do, causing the treatment to break down. In order to do so she would, in my view, have to work on her internal racism, as the second analyst had clearly done. If we cannot reach an accommodation with our internal racist it limits, in my view, the extent to which we can work effectively across cultural and racial boundaries.

Conclusion

In this paper I put forward the idea that internal racism exists in the mind in the form of an organised system of defences whose main function is to build in protection from primitive anxiety. Working from a clinical base I showed that it operates by setting up an internal racist organisation, which is deployed in three discernible steps, usually with lightning speed. First a real difference between subject and object is selected. Next, the subject, by means of projective identification, lodges an intolerable and unwanted part of itself in the object. Lastly, the internal racist sets about organising a set of relationships between self, object and relevant others, secondary to the original projection. The resulting network of relationships between people, each now containing different aspects of the self, appears as ordinary and unremarkable; and the existence of the racist structure is only revealed when the object behaves in an ordinary, rather than a scripted, way.

I think of the internal racist organisation as a normal pathological organisation. It is racist in that an arbitrary attribute of a person, usually identifying members of a specific out-group (e.g. skin colour, hair texture etc.), is chosen as the basis for massive projective identification. It is normal in three senses: statistical, normative and non-pathological. Statistically, I argued that everyone has an internal racist, citing as evidence the observation that a paralysis of functioning observed in the aftermath of a real racist attack on the streets in fact afflicts every cross-race encounter. As far as the second, normative aspect is concerned, it is usually members of socially endorsed out-groups who are targeted as the objects of racism, and social stereotypes inform the subject's views about the object. Lastly, I argued that internal racist functioning exists within a normal, rather than an ill, mind. Pathological organisation functioning is involved in that organised sets of extremely resilient defences are characteristic of the terrain of internal racism, which have all the hallmarks of a pathological organisation. Interventions incorporating an understanding of such defensive strategies, and the primitive anxieties they defend against, can paradoxically relieve the situation, though not without a struggle. This is because, while a pathological organisation occupies a large part of the energies of, say, the borderline patient, the racist organisation occurs in the normal mind, and it is the capacities of the normal mind that can help it pull through. Although anxiety that a catastrophe will result from facing internal racism is intense, the normal ego does, in fact, possess the resources to undertake such a struggle. Put another way, it is the organisation itself that generates intense anxiety in order to drive the subject into its arms for protection.

This latter point is important for the practising analyst. By emphasising its normality I mean to emphasise that it is possible for us to engage with our (own) racism, even though we would be inclined to resist this, and the process would of course be painful. None of us would easily own the fact that we would not want another human being to be him/herself, yet this is precisely what racist projection involves. It would probably be too much to expect this kind of self-scrutiny from the police officer in my example from the Stephen Lawrence case. However, if we bear in mind that our own personal analyses are meant to be a prelude for an on-going self-analysis that takes place throughout our career, then this is not an unreasonable expectation, especially for those clinicians who will be called upon to work with patients from cultural/ethnic backgrounds other than their own.

This work is bound to be highly sensitive and private, as it is not possible to tell from the outside who the object of our racism is or what form that racist object relationship takes. Externally, what is visible is only the paralysis, accompanied by political correctness, which indicates that we are not functioning optimally in the cross-cultural context. Kareem's second analyst illustrates how the work on his own inner racism – as a European during the Nazi era – had already taken place. Without this, I am suggesting, it would not have been possible for him to open up the inquiry into the relationship, in the patient's mind, between himself as a colonised Indian subject, and his English coloniser. By contrast, for the first analyst this was a no-go area.

Notes

1. A previous version of this chapter was published under the title 'Ethinsche Reinheit, Andersartigkeit und Angst: Das Modell des inneren Rassisus' in a special edition of *Psyche – Z Psychoanal 70*(9), 779–804. Stuttgart: Klett-Cotta, 2016. The paper is reprinted here in English with the kind permission of the publishers.
2. *The Guardian*, 8 December 2015. www.theguardian.com/world/2015/dec/08/germany-on-course-to-accept-one-million-refugees-in-2015. Accessed 12 April 2016.
3. I use the terms 'cross-race' and 'cross-culture' interchangeably, for reasons that I hope will become apparent.
4. The police officer visited the hospital where he was taken to find out whether she 'could have done more' (Norton-Taylor, 1999, p. 30).
5. I describe the details of this case more fully than I can here in Davids (2011).
6. For the sake of brevity I am not presenting a complete picture of Mr A's psychopathology here, for example, I do not consider the significance of his fear that his mother was dead. I give a fuller account in Davids (1995) and Davids (2011).
7. Both parents were described as seriously handicapped, each in their own way.
8. Much later he confirmed that, previously, he saw the therapist as an idealised mother.
9. A party of the far-right.
10. Stephen Lawrence was doing nothing more ordinary than waiting for a bus when he was murdered. I was doing nothing more ordinary than making an interpretation when my patient attacked me.

References

Dalal, F. (2002). *Race, Colour and the Processes of Racialization: New Perspectives from Psychoanalysis, Group Analysis and Sociology*. Hove and New York: Brunner-Routledge.

Davids, M.F. (1995). The management of projective identification in the treatment of a borderline psychotic patient. In J. Ellwood (ed.), *Psychosis: Understanding and Treatment* (pp. 162–80). London: Jessica Kingsley.

Davids, M.F. (2002). September 11th 2001: some thoughts on racism and religious prejudice as an obstacle. *British Journal of Psychotherapy*, *18*(3), 361–6.

Davids, M.F. (2006). Internal racism, anxiety and the world outside: Islamophobia post-9/11. *Organisational and Social Dynamics*, *6*(1), 63–85.

Davids, M.F. (2011). *Internal Racism: A Psychoanalytic Approach to Race and Difference*. Basingstoke: Palgrave Macmillan.

Freud, S. (1900). The Interpretation of Dreams. *Standard Edition, Vol. IV*. London: Hogarth Press.

Freud, S. (1917). Mourning and Melancholia. *Standard Edition*, *Vol. XIV* (pp. 237–58). London: Hogarth Press.

Hamer, F.H. (2002). Guards at the gate: race, resistance and psychic reality. *Journal of the American Psychoanalytic Association*, *50*(4), 1219–37.

Kareem, J. (1988). Outside in ... inside out ... Some considerations in inter-cultural psychotherapy. *Journal of Social Work Practice*, *3*(3), 57–71.

Kareem, J. (1992). The Nafsiyat Intercultural Therapy Centre: Ideas and experience in intercultural therapy. In J. Kareem and R. Littlewood (eds), *Intercultural Therapy: Themes, Interpretations and Practice*. Oxford: Blackwell Scientific Publications.

Leary, K. (2000). Racial enactments in dynamic treatment. *Psychoanalytic Dialogues, 10*(4), 639–53.

Macpherson, W. (1999). *A Summary of The Stephen Lawrence Inquiry: Report of an Inquiry by Sir William Macpherson of Cluny*. Norwich: HMSO. Retrieved from http://www.law.cf.ac.uk/tlru/Lawrence.pdf

Moss, D. (2001). On hating in the first person plural: thinking psychoanalytically about racism, homophobia and misogyny. *Journal of the American Psychoanalytic Association, 49*(4), 1315–34.

Norton-Taylor, R. (1999). *The Colour of Justice*. London: Oberon Books.

Perez Foster, R.M. (1996). What is a multicultural perspective for psychoanalysis? In R. Perez Foster, M. Moskowitz, and R.A. Javier (eds), *Reaching across Boundaries of Culture and Class: Widening the Scope of Psychotherapy* (pp. 3–20). Northvale, NJ and London: Jason Aronson.

Perez Foster, R.M., Moskowitz, M., and Javier, R.A. (1996). *Reaching Across Boundaries of Culture and Class: Widening the Scope of Psychotherapy*. Northvale, NJ and London: Jason Aronson.

Roland, A. (1996). *Cultural Pluralism and Psychoanalysis: The Asian and North American Experience*. New York and London: Routledge.

Rustin, M. (1991). Psychoanalysis, Racism and Anti-Racism. In *The Good Society and the Inner World*. London: Verso.

Sachs, W. (1937). *Black Hamlet* (with new introductions by Saul Dubow and Jacqueline Rose). Johannesburg: Witwatersrand University Press and Baltimore: Johns Hopkins University Press, 1996.

Sandler, J., and Sandler, A.-M. (1987). The past unconscious, the present unconscious and the vicissitudes of guilt. *International Journal of Psycho-Analysis, 68*(Pt 3), 331–41.

Schachter, J.S., and Butts, H.F. (1968). Transference and countertransference in interracial analyses. *Journal of the American Psychoanalytic Association, 16*(4), 792–808.

Steiner, J. (1987). The interplay between pathological organisations and the paranoid-schizoid and depressive positions. *International Journal of Psychoanalysis, 68*(Pt 1), 69–80.

Steiner, J. (1993). *Psychic Retreats: Pathological Organisations in Psychotic, Neurotic and Borderline Patients*. New Library of Psychoanalysis, 19, edited by E. Bott Spillius. London and New York: Routledge.

Thomas, L. (1992). Racism and psychotherapy: Working with racism in the consulting room – an analytical view. In J. Kareem and R. Littlewood (eds), *Intercultural Therapy: Themes, Interpretations and Practice*. Oxford: Blackwell Scientific Publications.

Chapter 2

Migration, loss and psychic retreat[1]

Kristin White

Moving in: moving away from the home country and settling into psychoanalysis

Each migration involves a very personal story of losing and finding oneself. The psychoanalysis of migration – the move from one country, language and culture to another – as I view it, is highly individual. Migration does not necessarily involve trauma or a crisis, even though it is trauma and crisis that we hear about again and again when the fate of refugees is discussed in the media today. Yet people migrate from one country to another or from one area of a country to another for a vast number of reasons, many of which have more to do with healthy development than trauma. We all agree, for example, that a young adult's wish to leave home is healthy and normal. And in our age of fast and comfortable transport that allows us to travel to faraway parts of the world with ease, it is no wonder that today's young adults travel further away when they begin to loosen their ties to the parental home. And many of these young people will take the opportunity to live abroad for some years. Some of them might then go on to meet a partner in the new country and settle down there and have children. Much can be gained and many new horizons can be met in the process of migration. And yet, something will always be *lost* when a person moves from one country to another. He might lose the close contact to his home country and his friends when he moves so far away. When he learns a new language, he might lose a part of his mother tongue in the process and find that he is no longer quite so up-to-date in his first language.

And these losses will inevitably be experienced in terms of each person's individual inner relationship to loss – as well as of course the mourning process that accompanies loss. It is the working through – or the avoidance – of such losses and mourning processes that can often be such a struggle in psychoanalysis with people who have experienced migration. The working through of such losses can indeed be a process that stretches across several generations, affecting the children and the grandchildren of the migrant (see Chapter 6 of this book).

The very personal nature of the effect of migration and speaking various languages is also described by Amati-Mehler, Argentieri and Canestri in their writings on speaking more than one language and psychoanalysis. They write of the polylingual (having had access to several languages since birth or in childhood which all function at the level of the mother tongue) and polylogical (organising different relationships within the self, according to different languages) person: 'There is ... no specificity of structure of the polylogical-polylingual subject, therefore, nor any peculiar pathology, or pathological predisposition that could perhaps affect a subject inhabited by more than one language' (Amati-Mehler, Argentieri and Canestri, 1993, p. 285).

I think that one can say the same of the migrant: there is no specificity and no particular pathology that we can attribute to those who have experienced migration: each one has his or her personal story and brings his or her own inner world with her into the experience of migration. Perhaps the only generalisation we can dare to make is the thought that just as it is difficult to leave home before we have grown up, it is very difficult to move away and find a new home if we are not at home in ourselves.

Mr A

A young English-speaking patient sought the help of psychoanalysis because of severe depression. He came to Germany to study the German language and literature. He wanted to be a writer but he was unable to find the words (in any language) nor to find a way of stringing them together. Worse still, not feeling at home in himself, he could not give his own words a home and was unable to feel attached to what he was writing. He seemed totally lost and was hardly able to function or even survive in the new (German) culture. He was living alone in an unheated, damp flat in the middle of a cold German winter and suffered from repeated chest infections. Therapy had to start by helping the patient to make contact to his basic needs so that he could put these in place. His very concrete, external needs, such as a place to live, kitchen equipment, furniture, food to eat or warm clothes for the winter could be addressed by way of a secure-base relationship that could help him to be in contact with neediness, also symbolically within the transference relationship, such as his need for friendship and understanding that was in constant conflict with his fear of abandonment and rejection. This patient seemed to have lost everything in the move to Germany and over the years this often reminded me of the migration of his own parents, who had both suffered the early deaths of their own parents and had had to manage alone with their siblings, standing on their own feet too early in life, migrating to a new country in the hope of a better financial future, but starting from nothing. It was as though my patient had to repeat the experience of building a home from nothing in a totally new environment.

In developmental terms, the experience of the loss of the mother over several generations was repeated in the migration experience as well as in the transference in the form of a child with a 'still-face' mother,[2] a severely depressed and 'dead' mother (Green, 1986) whom he was unable to bring to life, just as he was unable to bring his own words alive to be read or heard by a living object. In the transference the dead mother appeared as an unavailable object when the patient forgot his sessions or came at the wrong time, so that his analyst could not be available to him.

Symbolising loss

The loss involved in migration was for this patient not connected to a warm attachment to a home that he had once inhabited and which he could keep alive inside in the shape of the sadness of loss and idealised memories. Instead of the painful, but symbolised experience of *missing* his home, my patient concretely *missed* his sessions. He attempted to control the feeling of being abandoned by projecting it into me. *I* was the one who waited in vain for him to come back. For years, his psychoanalytic psychotherapy consisted of periods of missed sessions and even months in which he disappeared, obviously needing to experience again and again the reparative act when he returned and was able to find that the object had survived his destructive retreats.

In theoretical terms, we can think of my patient's difficulties externally in terms of attachment – the lack of an inner 'secure base' (Ainsworth et al., 1978; Bowlby, 1969; Holmes, 1993, 2010) and the development of an 'alien self' (Fonagy et al., 2002), Green's 'dead mother' (Green, 1975, 1986) or in Winnicottian terms, of the lack of survival of the destroyed object (Winnicott, [1969]1971). Whatever theoretical language we use, it is always about the early experience of the child and in particular his difficulties in navigating early experiences of separation and loss. From the point of view of *internal* experience, this is connected to the dominance of defensive organisations of the personality (Rosenfeld, 1971) and primitive defence mechanisms such as splitting and projective identification, in which misconceptions of the reality of separation and loss can arise (Money-Kyrle, 1968, 1971; Weiss, 2009).

Hanna Segal writes that when projective identifications are too concrete, there can be no symbolisation.

> It struck me in my work that concrete symbolism prevailed when projective identification was in ascendance. This also seemed logical. Symbolism is a tripartite relationship: the symbol, the object it symbolizes and the person for whom the symbol is the symbol of the object. In the absence of a person, there can be no symbol. That tripartite relationship does not hold when projective identification is in ascendance. The relevant part of the ego is identified with the object: there is not sufficient differentiation between the ego and the object itself, boundaries are lost, part of the ego is confused with the object, and the symbol

> which is a creation of the ego is confused with what is symbolized. It is only with the advent of the depressive position, the experience of separateness, separation and loss, that symbolic representation comes into play.
>
> (Segal, 1991, p. 38)

In the case of my patient, separation became a concrete action in the transference rather than a symbol. There was no triangular space to think about the missed sessions, nothing that could be mourned or missed, because he was simply not there. Any attempt by the analyst to address the issue when he returned was met by denial of the importance of the topic, surprise that the analyst should want to talk about it or it was turned around and made into the analyst's problem, not his own.

My patient had nothing to hold onto in the separation of migration because his depressed and 'dead' maternal object could not be sufficiently mourned, so that the internal parents had never come alive inside. The loss involved in migration was for this patient instead experienced as a loss of sense of self and meaning and he needed the help of analysis to build his inner world and to bring it to life over a long period of psychotherapy (see Weiss, 2009, pp. 116–32).

Some thoughts on migration through the ages: the myths of migration and their relevance to psychoanalysis

Grinberg and Grinberg (1984) have written about the three mythological stories that can help us to understand the inner dynamics of migration: the story of Oedipus, of the Tower of Babel and the story of Adam and Eve's exile from Paradise. Grinberg and Grinberg point out the similar movement in each of these myths: first there is a striving for knowledge, then punishment and exile:

> The myths of Eden, Babel and Oedipus illustrate and make more intelligible the conflict between those parts of the personality which seek knowledge and those which actively oppose this search. The conflict itself points to man's desire to 'migrate', to go beyond fixed borders in search of knowledge, wherever it may lie, while at the same time man has a tendency to put obstacles in his own path (prohibition). By so doing, he transforms the 'search migration' into an 'exile-expulsion-punishment migration', which gives rise to pain, confusion and isolation.
>
> (Grinberg and Grinberg, 1984, p. 4)

In the story of Oedipus, write Grinberg and Grinberg, there are numerous migrations: the first is the migration from Oedipus' parents to his adoptive parents as a baby. The second is his migration from his adoptive parents to Thebes in an attempt to avoid the fate that the Oracle had foretold, that he would kill his father and marry his mother. After the patricide and the incest are made known, there is a third migration when Oedipus is exiled to Colonos. Grinberg and Grinberg point out that it is curiosity and the wish to know the truth that is the drive behind the migrations of Oedipus:

> The Oedipus story can thus be seen as an example of the conflict inherent in human nature between the impulse to steal the father's most valued and desired possession, exposing oneself to punishment and exile, and the repression of that impulse.

According to Grinberg and Grinberg, in classical oedipal theory, the mother is considered the father's most valued possession and is the object of oedipal jealousy and rivalry. The other approach to the oedipal myth, and to the myth of Eden, holds that true knowledge, not the mother, is the object belonging exclusively to the father-God:

> Moses, who led the exodus of an enslaved people to the land of freedom, and who dared ascend the summit of Mount Sinai to seek knowledge of the Law, was punished by not being permitted to set foot in the Promised Land: he was allowed to see it only from afar before dying.
>
> (Grinberg and Grinberg, p. 7)

But what exactly is it that can turn the 'search' migration into an 'exile-expulsion' migration? The Grinbergs' suggestion is that it is man's 'tendency to put obstacles in his own path' in terms of 'prohibition'. The God in the myths of Babel and Paradise Lost and the Oracle in the Oedipus story are seen in terms of an inner super-ego power that puts obstacles in the path of desire, also the desire for knowledge.

But the drive for knowledge, to widen one's horizons through migration or to gain a greater knowledge of one's own self through the psychoanalytic process is not 'simply' a matter of overcoming a harsh and prohibiting super-ego, even though this remains one the core aims of the psychoanalytic process (Strachey, 1934). But it is not as simple as that: it is not just that we 'tend to put things in our way' or limit ourselves as Grinberg and Grinberg suggest, but much more that we often find it *hard to accept* the things that are put in our way, that is, our limitations. The decision to emigrate is very often connected to the longing for a better life, which is often an idealised wish to overcome limitations. Yet migration itself confronts us with our limitations: our weaknesses (for example, in the new language), our helplessness (for example, in the new culture), our neediness (for example, for support in the unknown world) and with loss (of all that we left behind). The inner work involved in migration is then not so much about overcoming a harsh and prohibiting super-ego but, on the contrary, dealing with an inner object that cannot bear the limitations and 'God-given' prohibitions.

The myths of Paradise Lost, Babel and Oedipus all point to man's struggle with limitations that are simply 'facts of life' (Money-Kyrle, 1971; Steiner, 1993; Weiss, 2009; White, 2013), that is, God-given, not man-made. These myths all make it very clear that it is foolhardy to try to be better than God, to question God's laws or to try to circumvent the wisdom from Delphi. According to Money-Kyrle (1971) and Steiner (1993), we have to recognise the *fact* of our dependence on others from birth onwards, the *fact* of the difference between the sexes and the passing of the generations and the *fact* that time passes and our lives do not go on for ever. It is these facts of life that man has a tendency not to recognise, leading to a *feeling* of punishment, exile, pain, confusion and isolation. These facts of life are in fact a very particular kind of knowledge – the knowledge of our limitations, that we are human and not gods, not omnipotent or omniscient. The painful knowledge of our broken inner worlds, of our helplessness and our fear.

If migration takes place against a backdrop of the denial of internal limitations, such as migrating to an exciting new country to escape the painful reality of oedipal exclusion, then this denial will be carried over into the experience of migration, turning it into what Grinberg and Grinberg describe as an 'exile-punishment' experience. The oedipal experience, for example, is then projected into the new country, which is experienced as exiling and punishing, rather than a place for new experiences and the expansion of knowledge. On the one hand, the experience of migration brings with it a tendency to make use of such primitive defence mechanisms as the projective identification that turns the new country into an exiling, punishing organisation. Yet when the migrant brings with him, in his internal world, a personality organisation involving denial and excessive projective identification, his experience of the new world and his ability to expand his knowledge in the new situation will be disturbed along the lines of his disturbed inner organisation. Migration is then experienced in the sense of non-knowledge or annihilating knowledge, Bion's -K (see also Joseph, 1983).

Two kinds of psychic retreat in the Oedipus story and their relationship to migration

In fact, the migrations and exiles in the story of Oedipus are not only related to a healthy striving for knowledge, but also for a striving for supreme superiority and omnipotence – to outdo the Sphinx and later omnipotent denial, when Oedipus is faced with a truth that he cannot bear to know.

John Steiner has connected the Oedipus myth to Money-Kyrle's 'facts of life' and has shown how Oedipus wanted at once to know and not to know these truths, pointing out how Oedipus gouged his eyes out in order not to see the truth, finally to be exiled to Colonos, where, according to Steiner, he could lead a life of omnipotent delusion and not-knowing. Oedipus on Colonos was unable to give up and mourn the loss of his omnipotent phantasy.

Steiner describes two very different states of mind that are shown in the two stages of the Oedipus story: when Oedipus gouges out his own eyes, he is also blinding himself to the unbearable truth of his anxiety, responsibility and guilt. Steiner relates this to the defence mechanism of 'turning a blind eye':

> Mechanisms such as '*turning a blind eye*' which keep facts conveniently out of sight and allow someone to know and not to know simultaneously can be highly pathological and lead to distortions and misrepresentations of the truth ... Oedipus adopts a state of mind which can be thought of as a psychic retreat from reality and a defence against anxiety and guilt.
>
> (Steiner, 1993, p. 129)

Steiner differentiates between this kind of retreat from anxiety and guilt and the 'retreat to omnipotence' (ibid., p. 129) in which Oedipus no longer feels shame and no longer tries to hide reality of his deeds. This is because he omnipotently denies his guilt and responsibility through his conviction that he had been a victim of Fate. That is, the gods were responsible. Of Oedipus at Colonos, Steiner writes:

> This kind of relationship to reality is based on a *retreat from truth to omnipotence* and is clearly very different from that of *turning a blind eye*. The retreat is one in which reality is dismissed and the organisation on which it is based is peopled with omnipotent figures who claim respect from their divinity and power. The truth does not have to be argued or justified and shame and guilt are inappropriate ... Here too we have a pathological organisation of the personality, but one organized at a more primitive level ... When they take on a paranoid grandiosity, as in Oedipus at Colonos, they seem to protect the individual from paranoid-schizoid disintegration and fragmentation.
>
> (Steiner, 1993, pp. 129–30)

Working through: migration as a psychic retreat

A psychic retreat from truth to omnipotence as defence against paranoid-schizoid fears

I think that the English patient described in the first part of this paper, Mr A, had moved to Germany as a retreat, defending against paranoid-schizoid disintegration. Moving away from his home country and speaking a different language had given him temporary relief from his fears, but when he entered psychotherapy he was clearly confused and hardly able to function or communicate. He had tried to hold onto some sort of contact to himself and the world with fleeting sexual contacts, but this gave him only temporary relief from his fears of breakdown. He was clearly suicidal and seemed to cling onto the hope of psychotherapy like a drowning person holding onto a floating branch. At the same time, the challenges and conflicts involved in *life* and in psychotherapy seemed to overwhelm him, so that he instead retreated into a near-to-death, drowning place (Segal, 1993). In his first session, he took one of my paper tissues and tore it up into little pieces, which he rolled up and strewed on the floor in front of him. I thought this was an apt description of his fragmented inner world from which he was trying to escape. Once he had his place in psychoanalysis however, and when he began to settle in, he took on a haughty, denigrating attitude, denying the helpless, needy part of his own self that had originally come for treatment. It was when he retreated into this state that he missed his sessions, turning the analyst into an unavailable object, but avoiding the feeling of missing this object himself. Instead, his *analyst* was left to helplessly wonder why he had disappeared yet again. Sometimes he cancelled a session and neglected to arrange a new one, sometimes then disappearing from analysis for months on end. Then he would turn up again, as needy and depressed as ever, but unable to reflect on his disappearance or neediness. Over the years, he attempted to embark on weekly psychotherapy as well as three-times-weekly psychoanalysis, but each time the same pattern emerged after a short time. He migrated in and out of analysis, as it were, controlling his depression by controlling the analytic process and projecting all feelings of helplessness into the analyst. He prevented any kind of integration between the states of being 'in' or 'out' of analysis as well as preventing the development of a third position where he might reflect on these states. He used to bring a bottle of water or food into the psychotherapy, offering the therapist to join him, thus creating the concrete illusion of two friends drinking tea together. In one of the phases when he had tried to use the couch, he brought a pad of notepaper and a pen, thus taking on the role of the psychoanalyst. In all of these situations, it was the separateness of an object that was at once so much needed and yet beyond his control that was feared the most.

It seemed to be the experience of being able to return repeatedly, of the analyst's tolerance of his claustro-agoraphobic (Rey, 1988) relationship pattern and the feeling of being understood in the little moments when he was able to emerge from the retreat to observe his inner self with the analyst that finally gave this patient enough containment for the fragmented parts of himself. At first, he used the phases of psychoanalysis and psychotherapy as an inner base to make steps in his life: he married, found a steady job and started a family. Yet he seemed to have hardly any feelings of connection to these relationships. Like the analyst, they were kept at an inner distance and were experienced as 'putting things into his life', rather than emotional relationships. In this way, he also kept these external objects under his control. It was only much later that he was able to embark on regular, once-a-week psychotherapy appointments in which he was gradually able to come to terms with the loss of the ideal object in the transference, that is, the object which was under his omnipotent control and to which he could might return on his own whim and who could free him from his loneliness and depression by being 'a friend with whom he could drink tea.' Painfully, he was able to begin to see himself as a patient and the analyst as a helpful, but separate object beyond his omnipotent control, who could help him with understanding and reflection rather than an extension of himself. Finally, he was able to negotiate a kind of ending in which the separation could be thought about, though with much pain, so that the migration 'into' and 'out of' analysis became something that could be joined by reflection and thus more integrated. It was of course not just chance that in the course of this process he was able to settle down in the new country, to feel at home in his family and externally as well as in the therapeutic process, no longer needed to use migration as a psychic retreat.

Psychic retreat as 'turning a blind eye' and defending against the fears of the depressive position

The losses involved in migration are both obvious losses such as the loss of the home country and the mother tongue, as well as more hidden, unresolved losses that may well be the conscious or unconscious reason to move away from the home country as well as to later embark on psychoanalytic treatment. These more hidden losses include the loss of a sense of self or the loss of meaning and purpose to life, which are a mark of deeper depressive states and personality disorders.

The psychic retreats of the kind described by Steiner involve splitting processes. As in the story of Oedipus, migration to another country might be used in order to uphold the split, moving literally away from the conflicts around limitations rather than resolving them. In this conception of splitting, it is not traumatic events, such as the migration itself, to which the individual has been subjected as a passive victim, that lead to a 'dissociative' kind of splitting, where the part of the personality connected with the trauma is cut off. The kind of splitting referred to here is splitting in the sense of disavowal, in which splitting is *actively* brought in by the individual to deal with an internal and external reality that is felt to be unbearable. As Steiner has described, this might be the kind of splitting where two versions of reality are upheld simultaneously, as in 'turning a blind eye', or a splitting process in which reality is defended against in an omnipotent and a deluded way. Migrating to a new country can be used in the service of both such defences.

Mrs B came to analysis as an older woman. She had spent her life moving away from conflicts that centred on her feelings of denigration and being second best. It seems that the start of this was the birth of her little sister when she was four years old. She had found it unbearable to be removed from the place of the most important and only child of her parents and had reacted with anger attacks that, as her parents reported with amusement, could be heard at the end of the street. Mrs B found a new way of being the first and best by excelling at school and going on to a grammar school of academic excellence. This distanced her increasingly from her family. She felt different – and better. But the experience of an elite university again put her in a place of second best – there were others around her now who were even better academically. Rather than accept this, she left her course unfinished and moved to a new place. Again and again in life, she moved away, often to new countries, when confronted with oedipal disappointments and the exile from the place 'at the top of mother's and father's favour'. This included leaving her marriage when she was confronted with the prospect of the triangular situation of a baby. In panic, she aborted the pregnancy and moved on. This pattern of exiling herself led to an increasing isolation and very little in the way of lasting contacts and friendships. She came to analysis when she felt physically too old to move away and start again. However, rather than retreating into an internal 'Colonos', a lonely psychic retreat, she was able – if sometimes unwillingly – to confront herself with Money-Kyrle's 'facts of life'. Bit by bit in the painful work of analysis, she was able to realise the importance of recognition from her friends and family and her dependence on them for her own sense of value. She was able to confront herself with the limitations of her own life and find a place for her life in the passing of the generations, picking up a long-lost thread of connection to her parents and visiting their graves. She had not known how they died or where they were buried as she had been abroad and lost the contact. As she re-discovered the inner contact in the course of analysis, the painful losses of all she had rejected, turned away from or missed out on had to be mourned. This was accompanied by intense feelings of guilt and regret (see also Steiner, 2011).

All the losses that Mrs B had suffered through her migrations had to be taken out of their inner hiding places and mourned. As Freud put it in the famous passage from 'Mourning and Melancholia': 'Each single one of the memories and situations of expectancy which demonstrate the libido's attachment to the lost object is met by the verdict of reality that the object no longer exists' (Freud, 1917, p. 255).

Moving out – the unsettling experience of moving away from analysis

After patients have settled into analysis and embarked on the long and intensive work of discovering understanding and being understood, there comes a time when both analyst and patient begin to realise that the work could now come to a close. The German health system, which usually pays for around 300–360 sessions of psychoanalysis, often precludes the inner work of coming to this realisation as the external pressure of the change to private payment of the sessions often leads to an ending that feels enforced from the outside. Despite all the wonderful advantages that the access to psychoanalysis for everybody brings, the fixed number of insurance-paid sessions can also sometimes 'save' both patient and analyst from the essential, but difficult inner work of the ending of psychoanalysis.

My experience of working with migrants has shown me that the work of separation at the end of analysis is often the point where, if all goes well, their internal and external feeling of 'home' is consciously re-addressed and consolidated. Many patients actually decide to move back to their home countries. Others are able to make the conscious decision to stay and build their home in Germany, rather than holding onto the begrudging feeling that paradise is always somewhere else in a place to which they themselves have no access. But the satisfaction of being able to be at home in society as well as in oneself requires the difficult work of separation and loss, not only the loss of the idealised 'paradise' to be found elsewhere, but also the loss of analysis itself, when it is clear that it is coming to an end. The longing for the perfect state at the end of analysis, an inner state in which all conflict is resolved and all the wished-for goals have been achieved, can turn the separation from the phantasy of an 'analytic paradise' into a painful struggle. The confrontation with the loss of analysis can then lead to another phase of retreat, and it is sometimes this stage of the analysis that gives the patient an important chance to discover previously hidden areas of their inner self in which they hold onto idealisations in a secret, conflict-free zone.

Steiner writes:

> Splitting is not restricted to the paranoid-schizoid position (Klein, 1935), and is resorted to again when the good object has been internalized as a whole object and ambivalent impulses towards it lead to depressive states in which the object is felt to be damaged, dying or dead and 'casts its shadow on the ego' (Freud, 1917). Attempts to possess and preserve the good object are part of the depressive position and lead to a renewal of splitting, this time to prevent the loss of the good object and protect it from attacks.
>
> The aim in this phase of the depressive position is to deny the reality of the loss of the object, and this state of mind is similar to that of the bereaved person in the early stages of mourning. In mourning it appears as a normal stage which needs to be passed through

> before the subsequent experience of acknowledgement of the loss can take place ...
>
> (Steiner, 1993, p. 33)

Mr A started to miss sessions again towards the end of his analysis, yet this phase of psychic retreat was essentially different from his previous retreats. He always informed the analyst of the sessions that would be missed and made sure that the next session was arranged, thus making sure that the analyst would not turn away too soon, despite his angry attacks. And the missed sessions could finally be spoken about and reflected on. In this phase of his analysis, he was able to overcome the retreat relatively quickly and to feel the underlying sadness and fear of depression in connection with the impending loss of his analysis. He sunk yet again into periods of deep depression and wondered whether he would manage without the help of the therapy. In the counter-transference, the therapist began to feel guilty about sticking to the arranged ending date, wondering whether the therapy might have to continue after all.

And yet, at the same time, Mr A let me know that he was now writing more freely and with enthusiasm. His paid work was obviously also going well and he was able to use his savings to buy property in the country where he was living, which he now considered to be his home. The inner work of mourning seemed to have set a creative process in motion through which he was able to find an inner an external secure base and to set up a home for himself in which he could express himself freely and creatively.

The more the losses that were experienced in migration can be experienced and mourned in the course of an analysis, the more creatively the new home can be filled with the expression of the creative self. As Hanna Segal has written:

> Every aspect of the object, every situation that has to be given up in the process of growing, gives rise to symbol formation ... In this view symbol formation is the outcome of loss, it is a creative work involving the pain and the whole work of mourning.
>
> (Segal, 1964, p. 76)

Notes

1. An earlier version of this chapter was published in *Zeitschrift für Individualpsychologie 43* (2018), 176–90, Göttingen: Vandenhoek und Ruprecht. The paper is reprinted here in English with the kind permission of the publishers.
2. The still-face experiment, which shows babies' reactions to non-mirroring mothers with a 'still face' can be seen as a YouTube video, introduced by Dr Edward Tronick, dated 30 November 2009. See also: Edward Tronick: *The Neurobehavioural and Socio-Emotional Development of Infants and Children*. New York: W.W. Norton & Co, 2007.

References

Ainsworth, M.D.S., Blehar, M.C., Waters, E., and Wall, S. (1978). *Patterns of Attachment: A Psychological Study of the Strange Situation*. Hillsdale, NJ: Erlbaum Associates.

Amati-Mehler, J., Argentieri, S., and Canestri, J. (1993). *Babel of the Unconscious: Mother Tongue and Foreign Languages in the Psychoanalytic Dimension*, trans. J. Whitelaw-Cucco. Madison, CT: International Universities Press.

Bowlby, J. (1969). *Attachment*. London: Hogarth Press.

Fonagy, P., Gergely, G., Jurist, E.L., and Target, M. (2002). *Affect Regulation, Mentalization and the Development of the Self*. New York: Other Press.

Freud, S. (1917). Mourning and Melancholia. *Standard Edition, Vol. XIV* (pp. 237–58). London: Hogarth Press.

Grinberg, L. and Grinberg, R. (1984). *Psychoanalytic Perspectives on Migration and Exile*. New Haven and London: Yale University Press.

Green, A. (1975). The analyst, symbolisation and absence in the analytic setting. *International Journal of Psychoanalysis*, *56*(1), 1–22.

Green, A. (1986). The Dead Mother. In *On Private Madness*. London: Karnac.

Holmes, J. (1993). *John Bowlby and Attachment Theory*. London: Routledge.

Holmes, J. (2010). *Exploring in Security: Towards an Attachment-Informed Psychoanalytic Psychotherapy*. London: Routledge.

Joseph, B. (1983). On understanding and not understanding: Some technical issues. *International Journal of Psychoanalysis*, *64*, 291–8. Reprinted in M. Feldman and E. Bott Spillius, *Psychic Equilibrium and Psychic Change: Selected Papers of Betty Joseph* (pp. 39–50). London: Routledge, 1989.

Klein, M. (1935). A contribution to the psychogenesis of manic-depressive states. *International Journal of Psychoanalysis*, *16*, 145–74.

Money-Kyrle, R. (1968). Cognitive development. *International Journal of Psychoanalysis*, *49*, 691–8.

Money-Kyrle, R. (1971). The aim of psychoanalysis. *International Journal of Psychoanalysis*, *52*, 103–6.

Reitman, J. (dir.) (2009). *Up in the Air* [motion picture]. Paramount, Los Angeles.

Rey, H. (1988). Schizoid Phenomena in the Borderline. In E. Bott-Spillius (ed.), *Melanie Klein Today. Vol. 1*. (pp. 203–29). London: Routledge.

Rosenfeld, H. (1971). A clinical approach to the psychoanalytic theory of the life and death instincts: An investigation into the aggressive aspects of narcissism. In J. Steiner (ed.), *Rosenfeld in Retrospect: Essays on his Clinical Influence* (pp. 116–30). London: Routledge.

Segal, H. (1964). *Introduction to the Work of Melanie Klein*. London: Karnac.

Segal, H. (1991). *Dream, Phantasy and Art*. London: Routledge.

Segal, H. (1993). On the clinical usefulness of the concept of the death instinct. *International Journal of Psychoanalysis*, *74*(Pt 1), 55–61.

Steiner, J. (1993). *Psychic Retreats*. London: Routledge.

Steiner, J. (2011). *Seeing and Being Seen*. London: Routledge.

Strachey, J. (1934). The nature of the therapeutic action of psycho-analysis. *International Journal of Psychoanalysis*, *15*, 127–59.

Tronick, E. (2007). *The Neurobehavioural and Socio-Emotional Development of Infants and Children*. New York: W.W. Norton & Co.

Weiss, H. (2009). *Das Labyrinth der Borderline-Kommunikation*. Stuttgart: Klett-Cotta.

Weiss, H. (2010). Perverse Verknüpfungen: Realitätsbezug und argumentative Struktur. *Jahrbuch der Psychoanalyse*, *60*, 101–21.

White, K. (2013). When migration is used as a defence against painful realities: some experiences of working with English-speaking patients in Germany. *Psychoanalytic Psychotherapy*, *27*(1), 41–59.

Winnicott, D.W. (1969). The use of an object and relating through identifications. In *Playing and Reality* (pp. 86–94). London: Routledge, 1971.

Chapter 3

Once around the world – the denial of traumatisation in the globalised post-modern world[1]

Monika Huff-Müller

The process of globalisation places an increasing demand on us to be able to change. In our current economy and society, this process of change is often imbued with positive connotations such as re-orientation and the development of new opportunities as a result of mobility and flexibility. Traumatic experiences caused by alienation and uprooting are often denied and repressed.

In psychotherapy, we can observe an increase in the trans-generational passing on of broken biographies and identity crises in the form of cumulative trauma that is not only due to flight and migration but also in cases of seemingly freely chosen mobility. Often ability of the psyche to transform itself has been overstrained in the process.

Typical trauma symptoms known from other historical contexts may then surface with all their destructiveness and demand a creative remodelling of the inner heritage with the help of psychoanalytic therapy. How can we use the knowledge of psychoanalysis in regard to formation of trauma?

Alongside our basic knowledge of psychoanalytic technique, we need to take our knowledge of the specific cultural and historical context into account in order to enable self-development and identity formation in such patients.

Introduction

In our work as psychotherapists, we often experience that uprooting and migration leave clear marks in the psyche of displaced persons. Broken lives and identities, the loss of social relations and social networks as well as the loss of relational systems and established bonds lead to mental strain and increased vulnerability. Enormous processes of adaptation are necessary which might be extremely stressful and may result in feelings of loss of control or even loss of meaning. We meet many such individuals when they seek psychotherapy.

We have become increasingly aware that the cultural, political and historical background must be considered in the case of traumatised refugees.

This background may also be important for the understanding of patients who have voluntarily left their home country and moved around in the post-modern world. What are the consequences of this for our psychoanalytic approach? In this chapter, I will examine different ways of dealing with the cultural, political and historical background of patients in the psychotherapy process.

If we reflect on our post-modern societies, mobility and emigration for economic reasons are no longer considered to be painful steps of separation and parting but as a natural course of action of the globalised human being. This perception presupposes a readiness for change and a flexibility in the individual, whereby mobility and emigration are perceived as a chance to acquire freedom or a search for happiness. However, it should be considered whether the richness of opportunities that is envisaged in our post-modern societies for those who leave their home countries behind, may in fact be a denial of uprooting in the sense of *Entheimatung*, that is, the loss of one's sense of home, or the loss of the homeland. Seen in this light, post-modern mobility might lead to an unconscious kind of traumatisation, in which patients take defensive measures against the expected mental pain and distress.

In patients who have experienced such post-modern developments, just as with refugees, one can observe a passing on of broken biographies and identities to the next generation in the form of transgenerational transmittance, even in cases of apparently freely chosen mobility. Often the transformation capability of the psyche will be strained for many generations. This often demands a creative transformation of the inner heritage through psychoanalytic therapy.

There is a danger of finding no way of coping with the phenomena of Entheimatung and the sense of foreignness within individual psychotherapies in post-modern times. Doing so the psychoanalyst would perhaps follow the often found denial and splitting off of the society as such.

The individual in post-modernism

Bovensiepen (2009) describes post-modernism as 'fleeting modernism'. The term 'fleeting' already points to 'fleeing'. He describes the 'generation global' as a generation which rarely has meaningful relationships. This generation does not experience relationships as an element of psychic development. In a pure network society, people swing on the one hand from a feeling of being related to everyone and everything due to being able to easily access global networks online. On the other hand, they experience a constant looming threat of losing relationships due to rapid changes in employment and location.

Conzen (2010) describes that in post-modernism the individual is degraded to an economic item, in which the 'subjugation of the individual under constantly changing conditions of his profitable exploitability is celebrated as the development of personality'. The self-image of post-modern man is characterised by self-determination and efficacy, in which feelings of impotence and heteronomy are hardly considered. His past seems to be condemned to be insignificant. Auchter (2004) remarks that post-modern man is 'unable to learn from experience, unable to use his memories'. Post-modern man is fixated on the here and now – he does not show any symptoms which means his unconsciousness appears to be empty. Machleidt (2008) describes that most migration stories are 'stories of successes. One often hopes for a new beginning and wants to escape from the 'entanglement with the history of one's own culture'. Langendorf (2009) points out that the post-modern system might result in a release of creativity, initiative and narcissistic self-realisation, yet at the same time it might lead to narcissistic self-exploitation and depressive fatigue as described by Ehrenberg (2004).

More than ever before, we follow an idea of the achievable in which foreignness is associated with the idea of unlimited mobility as a prerequisite of self-realisation and a narcissistic gratification. That it leads to uprooting, helplessness, powerlessness, confusion and narcissistic fragility, is often forgotten. Against this background Schneider (2009) describes a growing flexibility of the idea of identity with a compulsion for positivity and potentiality. This implies on the one hand a state of narcissistic superiority, while simultaneously leading to forms of narcissistic vulnerability and fear. This results in a development to a seemingly adolescent identity structure with a 'surplus of foreignness' which demands integration. Modern man is overstressed with these developmental tasks and reacts with defence and splitting.

The post-modern individual is considered to be the creator of his own self who is expected to achieve stability on his own without the need for relationships and ties. The fixation on achievement and success, overcompensation in the sense of Adler, is the attempt to gain recognition, to be a part of a new community and to find a new identity.

As psychoanalysts, however, we know that to remember is a necessary prerequisite in the constitution of identity. The post-modern stance of moving forward without a backward glance is highly problematic. Surely there is no standard type of the 'post-modern fugitive'; too varied are the individual journeys through life, experiences and conflicts in cultures and families.

Nevertheless, one does wonder whether those exhausted, 'homeless', highly successful members of our mobile society do not have some traits in common which then surface in the form of psychological symptoms during the challenges of stressful life events and crises. It could be that it is not only those who are clearly traumatised who carry losses and broken identities within themselves, but also those with apparently successful lives. A society which denies such consequences takes away the chances of the afflicted to understand and come to terms with their psychic problems and the chance to develop a proper self-understanding. One can describe identity as being constructed in the interaction of the individual with his or her culture. Denial and splitting of his own and his family's historical and cultural past leads to alienation and broken identities.

Migration, uprooting and the loss of the homeland

Ermann (2004) describes the severe psychic problems caused by uprooting and loss of the homeland in times of war. He points out that there is hardly any literature on the traumatisation and identity problems of the war generations. Mitscherlich had already described in *The Inability to Mourn* (1967) the problems of a whole generation in developing a feeling for the value of one's own self and the necessity to say goodbye to lost object relationships.

Nevertheless dealing with the psychic problems of the war generation came somewhat late. This generation has been too inconspicuous, free of symptoms and the resistance within society too strong to deal with this topic. Ermann describes the effects of the denial of mourning and loss on the German 'war children', those who were born between 1939 and 1945. The psychological development of these children is marked by early traumatisation due to their war experiences. He observes in this group a split awareness of their own biographies. Although they know about their past, the emotional awareness of their experience is split off and they are thus unable to understand themselves fully. They are unable to access the traumatisation that they have endured.

They lack both an understanding of the severity of the trauma and of the efforts that would have been necessary in order to cope with their experiences and the perception of their trauma. They do not perceive themselves as harmed or as traumatised victims nor are they seen as such by others. By way of transgenerational transmittance they served as a container of their parents' sufferings and sorrows. It was fundamentally important that they adapted to the new situation and fitted in. Thus they fulfilled the demands of post-war society, they were reasonable and hard-working. In the post-war era an aspiring, economically successful generation emerged. Later, it became apparent that many of those affected were not able to develop a feeling for their own needs and hardships. These feelings were split off and forms of alienation became visible. Identity-gaps developed. Unconsciously, they tried to carry out and fulfil the unspoken expectations of their failed parents. Caught up in the dynamics of parentification, they tried not to burden or blame anybody and became independent as soon as possible; they became competent and successful and in doing so healed the wound of the familial self. This was easily achieved on the basis of the German post-war 'economic miracle' and was generally accepted mode of being. Feelings of mourning, anxiety and emptiness were repressed in the process (Ermann, 2010).

Even today, we can observe in people who left their home countries for economic or business reasons, or in their children's generation, both feelings of alienation and an underlying sense of identity-loss as well as symptoms of depression, fear, guilt, distrust and the loss of self-esteem, even when the migration was apparently freely chosen.

Their own biography often remains foreign or even dispensable to them. They perceive their history as beginning at the point when they managed to participate in their 'new' societies successfully, as if there were no biography, neither for themselves nor for their parents or grandparents. Even in this post-modern generation, there are no inner images of their endured discontinuities, their changes of location or school. The effort that it took to come to terms with a new culture and language are also split off. They focus on functioning and adapting and try to take up the chances that are offered to them and use them successfully. Migration and uprooting are sometimes viewed as having a 'utopian moment' (Machleidt, 2008) which refers, in a rather one-sided way, only to ideas of a fresh start and success. However, people with this view of migration often develop states of confusion and emptiness in times of crisis and in threshold situations. For a long time they are successful and productive, adopt and adapt to new cultures and homelands, perform well at school, university or at their jobs. Yet suddenly they feel exhausted, experiencing their lives as empty and meaningless. The previously denied and split off aspects of their identity become relevant, now that they have entered a new culture. When I take the medical history of such patients, I often feel rushed, geographically and historically, as they tell me their life story. They speak of their past and their uprooting as though it were rather unobtrusive and the most natural thing in the world. Thus, I first have to feel the discontinuities in their biographies in my counter-transference. These patients are unable to understand this at first. The cultural, historical and geographical discontinuities are not perceived. Such discontinuities are confusing and threatening and consequently, defensive actions must be taken. As a result of these defence mechanisms there is no internal representation of the efforts they took to cope with their uprooting and the confrontation with feeling foreign. Thus, they often associate their efforts with the kind of exhaustion one might feel after having run a marathon.

The starting point of a therapy is usually that patients feel confused about their exhaustion and depression, including feelings of embarrassment and guilt. They are surprised by my interest in their biographies and their parents' and grandparents' lives. It had been the prime concern of these patients to look ahead and always to resume their normal functioning as soon as possible. They are surprised by my offer to look into their memories. In the course of their psychoanalysis, the numerous conflicts in their history and social and cultural environment come to light. I often feel pressure not to forget or omit anything. The 20th century was a century of dictatorships, war and expulsion. This has shaped biographies in which for example, one patient's grandparents had decided to settle in Russia, having escaped from Hitler, then endured a forced population transfer under Stalin and whose parents had decided to return to Germany after the fall of the Iron Curtain. Another patient had a Polish grandfather who had moved to France, where he met and married his Polish grandmother. The patient's mother then married an African man in Germany, where she had a daughter. Yet another patient was born in Germany and had a Chinese mother who had fled from persecution under Mao and met her German husband while working in Saudi Arabia. Over the generations, one can find cultural discontinuities, fractured biographies and deserted homelands which stand isolated without any relation to memory or emotion. There has been no chance of integration. Thus, the affected individuals are over-challenged, out of touch with their own identity and unable to develop a sense of authenticity. Whole continents and periods of life are mixed up. The exhausted patients feel confused as they experience symptoms of anxiety, depression, loss of meaning and isolation amidst an abundance of opportunities in their new lives.

Certain psycho-social competencies are necessary in order to hold onto a sense of self-continuity in the post-modern world, re-integrating the self after separations. After experiences of being uprooted, the affected person will be confronted with the conflicts in his or her biographical background and in this context feelings of isolation and meaninglessness might surface. This is in stark contrast to the perceived demand of the society to be successful. Defensive measures have to be taken against their own needs, wishes and uncertainty about being foreign. Ego functions are brought to the fore in order to protect one's own feelings of narcissistic grandiosity or those induced by one's family.

With regard to transgenerational transmittance: already in 1913, Freud had written in *Totem and Taboo*, 'We may assume that no generation is capable of concealing its more important psychic processes from the next' (Freud, 1913, p. 159). Past and present historical, social and cultural factors find their expression in the unconsciousness of the patient. They are part of a matrix of psychic processes which have to be taken into consideration within psychotherapy. Their family's images of re-orientation or desire to overcome trauma have left their mark on the patients. Unconsciously they are now intensively occupied with using their ego functions to cope with those fantasies and affects which do not derive from their own lives but in fact come from their parents' or society's fantasies and fictions. So the inner objects of the parents are absent and at the same time overwhelming. Just in the sense of how Lewinsky (2006) makes his protagonist say in the play *Just an Ordinary Jew*: 'You sometimes remember things that you did not experience at all'. This does not really fit with the claim of postmodernism, that the individual is able to create his reality again and again. This post-modern idea questions the value of remembering. Akhtar (1999) describes that migrants need a third individuation following Mahler's first and second individuation processes. The developmental task is a further challenge. Mahler describes the psychological birth of a human as a first individuation process which the child copes with through a succession of detachment, separation and individuation. The child is allowed to be afraid, to mourn, to separate and to enter the world. The second individuation is achieved in puberty in which the adolescent regresses and in doing so reviews and converts his self-image and that of his objects, in order to develop a mature identity. Following Akhtar, a third individuation is necessary in order to be able to cope with migration and develop a self of one's own. Probably, a further psychological birth must take place. Step by step, the patient explores this new world just like in the sub-phases of the psychic birth, in our psychotherapies. Volkan (1993) emphasises that many refugees cannot achieve this third individuation. This seems to be the case for uprooting in general.

In the analysis, these explorations of the world need the acceptance of feeling foreign and being foreign. Both the patient and the analyst have to deal with the foreignness.

We know that the experience and images of strong and safe attachments are necessary for individuation and separation. We also know that these processes need sheltering, mirroring and relatedness.

Dealing with *Entheimatung* (the loss of a sense of home) and foreignness in psychoanalysis

On the basis of the foregoing reflections the following question arises; how do we deal with the aspect of Entheimatung and foreignness in the psychoanalytic situation?

Auchter (2004) emphasises that in the process of psychoanalysis, a 'space for memories' is created best characterised by empathy, holding, interpersonal understanding and sustainable attachment. Remembering needs 'reliable conditions, the 'containing' presence of the other in order to allow biographical experiences to resurface which can only be endured and articulated in the presence of a witnessing other'. This task not only needs knowledge on unconscious processes, unconscious conflicts, early childhood development and attachments but also requires knowledge of social, cultural, historical and geographical conditions. With regard to the psychotherapeutic relationship, this implies that a constant perception of foreignness should be a constitutive element in the interaction between patient and analyst. In this context, Nedelmann criticises that the mainstream of psychoanalysis is fixated on early mother/child relationships and processes of transference. The patient however is dependent on the therapist's knowledge of his reality. Parin (cited in Nedelmann, 2005) points out that the analyst must recognise which factors of the macro sociality of a people, a class or a social stratum has influenced his analysand and still does so. Only with this knowledge can those parts of the ego be analysed which were formed or deformed by adjustment. Bruder-Bezzel (2005) also, opposes the notion that psychoanalysis is not competent with regard to social questions. And Bachhofen (2007) calls for the expansion of the psychoanalytic process to include a historical dimension. This means that as psychoanalysts, we must constantly reflect on the foreign reality and that we need to develop models to deal with that which is foreign to us, bearing in mind that we might never fully penetrate it.

There are in fact two elements of dealing with Entheimatung and foreignness in the psychoanalytic situation, which I will illustrate with the following case example.

The *first* is to perceive the foreignness and to realise it by mutual effort of therapist and patient and to incorporate it into therapy. This demands a thorough exploration of the patient's world, of his parents' and grandparents' biographies, including his geographical and historical background. This might sound obvious to some, but according to a study undertaken by Ermann (cited in Bachhofen, 2007), one finds hardly any relevant material regarding the parents and grandparents in the reports that accompany the applications to health insurance companies to cover the costs of therapy. At the same time, one needs to explore the foreign cultural circumstances and find a way of integrating these into therapy.

The *second* element of dealing with Entheimatung and foreignness in the psychoanalytic situation is to perceive the foreignness and to recognise it as a forming and constituting element within the psychotherapeutic relationship. This means that one allows the aspects of foreignness or being foreign to be a part of the psychotherapeutic relationship. Disconcertment is one of the elements that make up the psychotherapeutic relationship. The prerequisite is that the feeling of being foreign is recognised in the transference and counter-transference at an early stage.

Clinical illustration

In the following, I would like to report on a few aspects of a psychoanalytic psychotherapy of 300 sessions consisting of two to three sessions a week. In this therapy, there were many conflicts on a structural and intrapsychic level. An essential element of this therapy was the mutual effort to explore and accept the foreignness of the patient, the acknowledgement of her uprooting and the attempts to create a space for the foreignness in our psychoanalytical work.

In the initial consultation, the 28-year-old patient reported feelings of depression, meaninglessness and isolation. Although she excelled in her studies, she was unable to finish her degree and this had plunged her into a severe crisis. She could not concentrate on her work. It was clear that she was very worried about this and she was full of self-contempt. She was extremely anxious and exhausted. As an intelligent and efficient student, she was used to being highly esteemed by her professors. At our initial consultation, the extremely slim and petite woman with Asian features presented as intelligent, differentiated and bright.

She lived with a friend who was also hard-working, so that their relationship was somewhat distanced, yet it nevertheless had a stabilising effect on her. She had never lived on her own and she could not be alone, she claimed. From the age of 12 she had eaten as little as possible, she told me, as if it were the most natural thing in the world and at present she had reduced her daily rations further and her bulimic episodes had become more severe which increasingly exhausted her. Since she had moved away from home at the age of 17, she had tried to eat nothing at all. Now she wanted to rid herself of her hunger, yet she was not able to take care of herself. When she told me that her daily ration consisted of a handful of nuts and two slices of bread, the remark: 'That's like a ration in a labour camp' escaped me. We were alarmed: the remark was disconcerting for both of us: We were disconcerted with each other. We agreed that we would try to understand these feelings of disconcertment. We looked into the associations surrounding the labour camp image and it was then that I approached her concerning her Asian appearance, her life story and that of her parents. Their narratives came to light bit by bit and the connections to the labour camp image became clear. On one hand the element of foreignness became an aspect of our relationship and on the other hand the element of foreignness invited us to explore it.

As a Chinese nurse, her mother met the patient's German father in Saudi Arabia where both had been working due to the better job prospects. After one month, her mother found herself pregnant. The father, afraid of repressions in a Muslim country, took her to Germany where he thought there were better conditions for raising a family. However, she was rejected by her Bavarian parents-in-law, which I could easily imagine, as we both had images and ideas about rural life in Bavaria in the 1980s and the reluctance there to accept foreigners. What life was like in Saudi Arabia for German engineers and Asian nurses only became apparent later after having made some enquiries in books and the internet. Due to pressure from her in-laws, the mother left the father while she was pregnant and tried to return to China. There her family, who had been fleeing from persecution in the 1940s, urged her to return to Germany where they felt that she would have better chances. The fictions of the mother and her relatives were characterised by the idea that support, safety and choices in life could be found somewhere else where there they could be free from the threat of rejection or repression – the utopia of a new beginning. Thus, the mother returned to Germany and the patient was raised by her single mother. She felt rejected and unwanted and was confronted at an early stage with the rejection and violence of her aggressive, overwhelmed mother while her father denied paternity and failed to establish any contact with her. During her stays in China, she was beaten in public, a customary practice so she claimed. In Germany she was beaten only in the privacy of their flat, particularly when she failed to obey without question. At kindergarten and school, she was successful and at the top of her class and was able to find self-confidence in her academic achievements. Yet she was hardly able to access her psychological distress and the emotional impact of her life experiences was foreign for her. Her starvation diet was an expression both of her desire for independence (not to need anything or anybody) and an expression of her self-contempt as she tried to make herself thin in keeping with her picture of the thin and petite Chinese person. Again and again, we referred back to historical and cultural pieces of information during her psychotherapy, so that her foreignness found a proper space as our mutual knowledge about her grandparents' and parents' realities grew. We were able to find words for the influence these conditions had on the life and the mental images of the patient.

The patient remembered how she had always felt divided between her Chinese and German identity, each of which was despised in the other country respectively. In China she was the Nazi child, in Germany the Chinese brat. She felt the pressure to produce outstanding achievements and be successful and she hoped to gain this by being perfect for both cultures.

Culturally, different concepts of the family also played a role. They, too, were looked into, according to the motto that psychoanalysis is a sophisticated game of hide-and-seek in which it is 'joy to be hidden but disaster not to be found' (Winnicott, 1965, p. 186).

For a long time the patient tried in vain to develop a secure sense of self by adapting to her mother's ideals and prayed every night to become a good daughter. She felt the destructive force of her punitive mother but could not question it. Here, the Chinese principle of the veneration of the elders was at work. It was painful for her to remember how – at the age of five – her mother left her for days on end at a Chinese restaurant whose landlords she hardly knew. Yet, she demanded of herself that she endure separations without complaining. She could feel that this was too much for her, but Chinese parental objects should not be called into question. Later, the patient became aware of the abandonment by her mother, which had been passed down from mother to daughter. She was then able to understand the specific transgenerational trauma of her Chinese family.

In her therapy, many questions were raised, such as, 'What are Chinese mothers allowed to do?' 'What are German mothers allowed to do?' and 'Is it a relevant question to consider the needs of a child?' Here a relationship came into being in which the German and foreign realities gained significance. A differentiated modified approach was necessary to recognise the cultural differences, to describe them, to explain them, and to separate them from the traumatic family history.

At the same time, I tried to introduce my knowledge of human development into her therapy for example by giving her information about early mother-child-relationships, which was a completely foreign notion for this Asian patient. In so doing, a container for the suffering of the patient could be formed. In the course of her therapy, the patient became more and more able to differentiate between the caring and protecting inner voices and those that tried to undermine and crush her. She began to take care of herself and she was able to eat more. Now she ate some nuts and a small jar of baby food.

Later on, it helped the patient to externalise her internal voices by writing down words and phrases and putting the notes into a box that was covered in Chinese symbols. Her affect regulation was at this point still rudimentary. In therapy, a potential space could be established in which her affects could find expression, so that containment and mentalisation became possible.

Later, when the patient felt her pain and despair and was often tearful in her sessions, she came to terms with her suffering and history and probably with her parents' and grandparents' history too by putting her wet tissues behind a clay screen in my office which I had bought on a trip to China. She called this her Chinese wailing wall and her tissues stayed there for about three months until she decided that she had mourned long enough. Here one can see again the constituting element of foreignness, which was held in the therapeutic potential space for months. I was able to allow the patient to make use of me, which helped her to deal with the family trauma.

Thus it became possible to consider her relationship to her mother in a new way and she became aware of her own desolation and the inability of her mother to take care of her – probably having been traumatised herself. In this phase it became obvious again and again how much support the patient needed and how empty she felt inwardly. With my support, the patient started to look for caring structures, for example, among friends or by contacting colleagues. Chiefly, I explained her affects, her emotions and explained 'her world' to the patient. Through the processes of mentalisation the patient was able to make true progress and was increasingly able to rely on her potential and her resources. She started to sympathise with both *her Chinese and her German* side.

The therapeutic techniques of mirroring and clarification led to a maturing of her ego-structures which had previously been weak. She gradually became more able to understand herself and others. The patient coped better with tensions and learned to anticipate these. Self-harming behaviour such as self-inflicted cutting became less frequent and the patient tried to find other ways of expressing herself.

It was my task to articulate this, to put it into words and to relate it to her experiences, her past and her unconscious. However, when her cold and traumatised mother once visited her, the patient entered into a state of crisis, in which both her old destructive conflict and the transgenerational conflict were reactivated. The patient felt again the inner pressure to be the perfect Chinese daughter and was afraid of failing miserably. When a Chinese meal did not turn out well, she angrily kicked a chair and broke her foot; later on in a similar situation, she broke her hand. The aggressive relational attacks by her mother with the unpredictable and disapproving parental injunctions resulted in a feeling of uncertainty in her and in an insufficient self-constancy and object constancy. At first, I was not available as a transitional object for her, but was more of an object to aid her development, with the aim of forming a structure on which she could cope with conflicts and come to terms with them. The main aim was to reduce their harmful and damaging influences. She was unable to separate from her mother. The Western idea of autonomy did not fit in with the internal images of the Chinese patient.

Her only mode was either destruction of herself (auto aggression) or of the object (breaking off relationships). She considered herself to be her mother's puppet and completely at her mercy. When we reconstructed her mother's escape route from Taiwan to Saudi Arabia via Bavaria to West Germany by means of an atlas, the patient could come into contact with her mother's uprootedness; she developed a sense of her mother thinking not only of herself but also of the patient, despite all the violence. She recognised that her mother was both victim and perpetrator. She was able to free herself from the compulsion to empathise with her mother. In so doing, she was able to begin her own biography. In her analysis, the idea of being home could be accepted for the first time and thus the foreignness too found a place. In this phase of the therapy, the patient's weight stabilised. The patient could see the connection between her weight and her internal conflicts. She allowed herself to be aware of her desire for safe attachments and individual self-esteem, which were forbidden desires within the Chinese culture of her traumatised mother. She needed the support of a mentalising function to make contact with these feelings. She wrote down the insights that she had gained in her therapeutic sessions on posters and hung them in her flat: 'I am accepted by the world', 'I am a valuable person, even without my accomplishments', 'There are people who are important to me and to whom I feel related'. Thus she developed from a silent child into a speaking adult. The process of mentalisation needed the affective and emotional experience of a safe attachment, which amongst other aspects, included the exploration of her broken past. The safe attachments developed in a mutual space of exploration and remembering.

I was repeatedly worried about the patient's weight which was checked once a month by her GP. At the same time, I had to ask myself whether our ideas of body and weight apply equally to the Chinese and the German cultures. Is the BMI valid for Chinese people? We had to find this out together. The patient started to accept that she needed food, but she also began to accept that she hungered after nourishment, warmth, stability and relationships. She began to understand that she could take action to achieve these. She realised now that certain things were good for her. The prime task in therapy was to put this into words and to clarify it. It took a long time before the patient was able to eat a warm meal. At the end of her therapy, her favourite dishes were Chinese soup and German butter cream cake.

A further aspect in this context was her internal conflict between autonomy and dependence.

Her desire to be taken care of on the one hand and her ideal of needing no food, of not being hungry on the other hand, was meaningful in this context. In her anorexia, the patient staged her lack of early object-experience and simultaneously her desire to be self-sufficient. The patient remembered that in puberty she had wanted to leave her family and so when she was 17 she travelled to the US, hoping to find a new identity there. The utopian element in migration and uprooting was apparent in this move. In the US she suffered a mental breakdown and then attempted to compensate for her isolation and despair by taking drugs (cannabis, cocaine) and engaging in a love-affair as a manic defence. When this adolescent love-affair failed, she made a suicide attempt under the influence of drugs and was then committed to psychiatric care. Because of this crisis she had to break off her stay in the US, which she continued to consider as a failure. During her stay in the US, the patient experienced a failure of her phantasy of self-sufficiency, which led to her breakdown. Her mother and her German stepfather, whom her mother had married when the patient was eight years old, reacted to this crisis with denial so she received no psychotherapeutic treatment at that time. On her return to Germany she fell in love with a German student, moved away with him in the 12th grade and finished school one year later in a new city. The impending failure at university that had been caused by exhaustion and fear when the therapy began, reminded the patient of the collapse of her American dream. Until then, the patient had not been able to realise that she had found a new home and identity in her studies in which she experienced resonance, support and stimulation. Her choice of subjects – German and English – (I do not remember ever having a more eloquent patient) – can surely be seen as an attempt to find her identity. Interestingly, her special topic of research was a poet who had been persecuted by the Nazis. When she was approaching the end of her studies, she realised the impending loss of structure. Leaving the protection of her university which had become her surrogate home and family triggered feelings of fear and anxiety. For quite a long time it remained unclear whether she would be able to take her final exams, as the end of her studies once again meant the loss of a home and another experience of uprooting.

The patient only knew the family injunction: 'Go somewhere else without looking back!'. Confronted with the end of her studies, the patient felt the imminent loss. In her analysis, she became increasingly aware of the fact that she needed relationships and an internal home. While her contacts until then had seemed to be without a clear purpose and rather indiscriminate, she now began to perceive the different possibilities of contacts and relationships. She now freed herself from the phantasy of having no real home and felt safe enough to investigate her uprooting and her roots. There was now a before and after for the patient. She was rooted in time. On the basis of this assurance the patient was able to end her studies successfully.

With this topic in mind, it is perhaps also important to mention how we dealt with the separations in analysis due to my holidays. The patient did not take any holidays during therapy. Due to the above mentioned processes of separation and individuation and her background of uprooting, violence and insecure attachment, I took a modified approach in dealing with my absences in the course of the therapy. Travel routes and maps of the countries I visited were allowed to play a role in the therapy. The patient initially reacted with strong feelings of fear when I informed her of my first holiday. She felt helpless and powerless. To combat this, we studied my foreign holiday destinations together. The travel route during my three-week absence was marked on a map and this helped the patient to survive psychologically. Before my second holiday, the patient developed a schedule for my absence and wanted to know where I would be travelling. When one year later a third separation was coming up, she packed an 'emergency case' together with me which she filled with different transitional objects, for example, a stone from my practice, the phone number of my colleague and the emergency number of a psychiatric clinic. Before my last holiday she chose a different form. We made a list of all her friends whom she could contact. Furthermore, she could speak on my answerphone which she used as a container for feelings she could not bear. Thus the patient was able to find ways of coping with feelings of emptiness and self-contempt during the separations. Sometimes it was necessary for the patient to be able to phone me in order to feel safe and to care for herself, for example when writing her MA thesis, to remember to eat a warm meal or to come to terms with a conflict with her friend. This led to a positive transference in which she perceived her therapist as an object that is present and interested in everything, both the known and the unknown, foreign things, both in the past and in the future. All this helped to restore her symbolising capability.

Finally, I would like to describe the following dream that the patient dreamt towards the end of her therapy: The therapist had invited her and her parents for breakfast. It was a German breakfast arranged like her friend always arranged it. Her mother ignored everything that was German, her father complained because of the tomatoes. Suddenly the plates transformed into Chinese dishes. When her parents showed no reaction whatsoever, the patient became very angry and started to shout at them.

There is much that one could mention about this dream. It describes the wish to break the silence and to face the psychological, social, cultural and historical elements of her identity and it is also an expression of the anger towards her parents who could not deal with their own trauma but instead passed it on to her.

At the end of the therapy the patient married and wanted to become pregnant. Despite many obstacles, she quickly became pregnant. After the birth of her child she visited me with her four-week-old daughter in my practice, and once again the foreign element shaped our meeting. When I pointed out the beautiful ears of the child, the patient remarked that the ears were bent, so she planned to tape them. When I looked at her in a rather disconcerted way, we both exclaimed at the same time: '*No Chinese methods!*'

In this therapy, 'Chinese methods' had been a symbol for all the trauma in the past of her family and so I added: '... not now, not here!'

Note

1. Translated by Maria König, Aachen and Kristin White, Berlin. This chapter is a slightly modified version of a paper published in *Zeitschrift für Individualpsychologie, 42* (2017), 229–43. Göttingen: Vandenhoek und Ruprecht, and is reprinted here in English with the kind permission of the publishers.

References

Akhtar, S. (1999). *Immigration and Identity: Turmoil, Treatment and Transformation.* Northvale, NJ: Jason Aronson.

Auchter, T. (2004). Die Fähigkeit zu erinnern und die Unfähigkeit zu erinnern. In Auchter, T. and Schlagheck, M. (eds), *Theologie und Psychologie im Dialog über Erinnern und Vergessen.* Paderborn: Bonifatius Verlag.

Bachhofen, A. (2007). Trauma und Transgenerationalität. *Forum der Psychoanalyse, 23*(3), 254–65.

Bovensiepen, G. (2009). Moderne Entwicklungstheorien – Eine Antwort auf die Objektflüchtigkeit in einer globalisierten Welt? In Münch, K., Munz, D., and Springer, A. (eds), *Die Fähigkeit, allein zu sein.* Gießen: Psychosozial Verlag.

Bruder-Bezzel, A. (2005). Wirtschaftliche und soziale Fragen können hier nicht zur Behandlung kommen. Kann die Psychoanalyse mit der Realität der Arbeitslosigkeit umgehen? In Springer, A., Münch, K. and Munz, D. (eds), *Psychoanalyse heute.* Gießen: Psychosozial-Verlag.

Conzen, P. (2010). Erik H. Erikson – Pionier der psychoanalytischen Identitätstheorie. *Forum der Psychoanalyse, 26*(4), 389–411.

Ehrenberg, A. (2004). *Das erschöpfte Selbst.* Frankfurt am Main: Campus.

Ermann, M. (2004). Wir Kriegskinder. *Forum der Psychoanalyse, 20*(2), 226–39.

Ermann, M. (2010). Verdeckte Spuren deutscher Geschichte. *Forum der Psychoanalyse, 26*(4), 313–24.

Freud, S. (1913). Totem and Taboo. *Standard Edition, Vol. VIII* (pp. vii–162). London: Hogarth Press.

Langendorf, U. (2009). Eiszeit-Vereinsamungsangst durch Arbeitsverlust. In Münch, K., Munz, D., and Springer, A. (eds), *Die Fähigkeit, allein zu sein.* Gießen: Psychosozial Verlag.

Lewinsky, C. (2006). *Ein ganz gewöhnlicher Jude*. Gelesen von Ben Becker Hörbuch-Roman: Hoffmann & Campe.

Machleidt, W. (2008). Kränkung und psychische Krankheit. In Heise, T. (ed.), *Von Gemeinsamkeiten und Unterschieden*. Berlin. VWB.

Mahler, M. (1998). *Symbiose und Individuation*. Stuttgart: Klett-Cotta.

Mitscherlich, A. and Mitscherlich, M. ([1967]1988). *Die Unfähigkeit zu trauern*. 20th edition. München: R. Piper and Co. [English edition, *The Inability to Mourn: Principles of Collective Behaviour*. New York: Grove Press, 1975].

Nedelmann, C. (2005). Zur Psychoanalyse der Entfremdung. *Forum der Psychoanalyse*, *21*, 323–32.

Schneider, G. (2009). Identität und die Ambivalenz gegenüber Fremdem. *Forum der Psychoanalyse*, *25*(1), 3–13.

Volkan, V.D. (1993). Immigrants and refugees: A psychoanalytic perspective. *Mind and Human Interaction*, *4*, 63–9.

Winnicott, D.W. (1965). Communicating and not communicating leading to a study of certain opposites. In *The Maturational Process and the Facilitating Environment* (pp. 179–92). London: Hogarth Press.

Part II

Languages, symbols and internal space

Learning foreign languages can open the door to a closer contact to the world. Yet foreign languages can also be used as hiding places to protect the ideal self and the ideal object.

Discussing the development of symbolisation and the depressive position, Hanna Segal has written about the importance of containment for the development of symbolisation in analysis:

> The psychoanalytic setting, with its regularity of time and place, the supporting couch, and so on, is one of the factors in this containment. But the crucial factor is the analyst's understanding. It is when the patient feels understood that he feels that what he projected into the analyst's mind can be processed by that mind. He can then feel mentally contained. When, for external or internal reasons, this benign interchange does not happen its place is taken by a relation between the container and the contained which is mutually destructive or denuding.
>
> (Segal 1991, p. 53)

When people move from one country and language to another, they sometimes consciously or unconsciously hide the uncontained and fragmented parts of themselves behind the foreign language and the fact of being a foreigner. This might even be a conscious process. An English-speaking patient who had moved from her home country to Germany for example, spoke openly about how she felt more comfortable in the foreign country and language (which she also spoke fluently) than in her home country, because she thought that the parts of herself which she experienced as 'weird' were seen to be linguistic errors rather than personal deficiencies.

More often, the hidden, uncontained part of the personality is unconscious and can only be discovered in the process of analysis. And it is this hidden part which needs to be understood so that the patient can experience containment through a feeling of being understood, thus feeling more integrated, both within himself and in his new environment.

Amati-Mehler, Argentieri and Canestri have written about splitting in the context of languages and migration. They distinguish between a kind of bi-lingualism in which languages can be used playfully from birth or in childhood and the bi- or multi-lingualism of the 'polyglot', who has learned different languages at later stages of life and psycholinguistic development so that there may be a less playful, more rigid exchange between the languages. They quote various literary authors who experience their bi-lingualism in terms of splitting. One example is the writer and essayist Tzvetan Todorov (1985), who wrote,

> Each language could be sufficient to the totality of my experience, and neither of them was clearly subordinate to the other ... One of these two lives had to be a dream ... Dreams and madness are/only a way of reacting to the schizophrenic situation itself ... The incoherence of the spirit is perfectly coherent with the incoherence of the world.
>
> (Todorov, p. 25, quoted in Amati-Mehler, Argentieri and Canestri, 1993, p. 62).

These experiences of splitting can be contrasted with Amati-Mehler, Argentieri and Canestri's description of polylinguals who have learned from an early age to include playing with languages in their experience of play. They write of the

> everyday dimension where we can perceive calmer and more serene signs of polylogical functioning ... It seems as though a spontaneous linguistic geometry is taking place, aimed not so much as separating but at maintaining the bonds as privileged channels along which the various languages convey constellations of affects and of the principal relational modalities.
>
> (Amati-Mehler, Argentieri and Canestri. p. 287)

References

Amati-Mehler, J., Argentieri, S., and Canestri, J. (1993). *The Babel of the Unconscious: Mother Tongue and Foreign Languages in the Psychoanalytic Dimension*. Madison, CT: International Universities Press.

Segal, H. (1991). *Dream, Phantasy and Art*. Abingdon: Routledge.

Todorov, T. (1985). Bilinguisme, dialogisme et schizophrenie. In A. Bennani, A. Bounfour, F. Cheng et al. (eds), *Du bilinguisme*. Paris: Éditions Denöel.

Chapter 4

Romania and its unresolved mourning[1]

Ilany Kogan

In this chapter, I explore the phenomenon of delayed mourning due to migration, both on an individual level and on a societal level. While migration is the more general term, strictly speaking, to *emigrate* means to leave one's country and to *immigrate is* 'to come to a country of which one is not a native, for the purpose of permanent residence' (Stein and Urdang, 1968). I will first describe the phenomenon of delayed mourning for primary objects due to migration on an individual level, basing it on a therapeutic encounter between a patient who had recently emigrated from Romania to Israel and a Romanian-born Israeli analyst. I will then examine the unresolved mourning of Romanian society, which was transplanted from one culture to another by means of its transition from a Communist dictatorship to the post-Communist era – another form of migration. This unresolved mourning was also expressed through the longing of many Romanians for the infamous leader, Nicolae Ceausescu, who functioned as a mental representation of a father figure. The longing is a clear indication that his followers internalised his image and therefore found it difficult to change their identification with this leader, even long after he had been executed. In Romania, the influence of Nicolae Ceausescu continued to have far-reaching effects years after his execution on 25 December 1989 (Volkan, 1998).

An immigrant patient and an analyst of the same national origin

Anna, a young doctor specialising in psychiatry, had emigrated from Romania to Israel several months before she was referred to me. Anna had completed her medical studies in Bucharest and was now completing her internship in a psychiatric hospital in Israel.

In the first session, Anna told me that she was referred to me by the senior psychiatrist of the locked ward where she was working. This psychiatrist, a woman who had also emigrated from Romania to Israel many years ago, befriended her and tried to help Anna adjust to her new country. Anna had been feeling quite depressed since her immigration to Israel and she derived strength from their friendship. Lately, their conversations had revolved around having children, since Anna, although married for seven years, had not yet tried to conceive a child. These conversations aroused much sadness in Anna, who claimed that she was not fit to have children of her own. It was in response to this that the friend suggested the possibility of therapy. Anna accepted the idea with the request that the therapist speak her own mother tongue. The psychiatrist friend then referred her to me.

Although initially hesitant about conducting analysis in Romanian because of my lack of fluency in the professional terminology of the language (I had emigrated from Romania as a child), I agreed to do it, because it is nonetheless my mother tongue, and I thought that it could be an enriching experience for us both.

Anna was an attractive woman in her early thirties. She had brown hair and brown eyes, an expressive face, and a feminine demeanour. Anna spoke to me in Romanian, and I was impressed by her fluency in the language.

From the very start of therapy, using my mother tongue had a strong emotional impact on me. I felt excited yet somewhat intimidated. My mastery of the Romanian language is relatively good, so I am often told. But relative to whom? I now asked myself this question while listening to Anna. Relative to a twelve-year-old child, the age at which I had illegally emigrated from Romania together with my parents, I silently answered myself. I had not forgotten the language, since it was the language I had spoken at home with my parents in Israel throughout my adolescence, but I had never acquired a more sophisticated Romanian in adulthood.

I was aware that my feeling of intimidation stemmed from a very deep personal experience from childhood that echoed inside me from our first encounters. The Romanian language represented a world of purely private experiences for me. The story in the family was that although my parents spoke German at home, I preferred to speak Romanian, which I had learned from my nanny. The nanny was a devoted Christian Adventist who had taken care of me as a child and had showered me with love.

Although I have conducted analyses in foreign languages that I learned to speak later in life, nothing was further from my professional world than the language of my childhood and adolescence. Would I be able to conduct analysis in this language, so distant from my professional work? It became clear to me that by accepting my patient's terms, I had lost the asymmetry necessary for a therapeutic relationship (Zac de Filc, 1992). Moreover, my simple, unsophisticated language placed me in the position of a child, especially when confronted with the elegant language of my 'grown-up' patient. I began to wonder whether this unusual situation, in which the therapist finds him- or herself linguistically disadvantaged, with all its emotional implications, might not have a negative effect on the treatment. I asked myself, What had I compromised by accepting, albeit with some misgivings, my patient's request? On the other hand, didn't my patient have a right to treatment, in spite of being a new immigrant to this country and not having command of the local language? Did I have the right to condemn her to silence and a childless fate, without giving her the opportunity to struggle against it?

I will not describe the entire course of this long and complex analysis. Instead, I will focus upon Anna's identity problem, which had become even more pronounced as a result of her immigration to Israel. I will then deal with the working through of her incomplete mourning for her parents, the postponement of which had been aggravated by her immigration.

From the beginning of her treatment, I was aware of Anna's nostalgia for the country she had left behind. Anna's memories centred more on places than on people. She recalled the houses, cafés, street corners, hills and countryside of her homeland. During her sessions, my office was filled with the colours, sounds, and smells of places familiar to both of us from our childhoods. This made me understand why Anna wanted to talk to me in her mother tongue. She wanted to share her very early experiences of a place that she hoped was familiar to me from my own childhood. Anna was looking for a special kind of understanding.

The therapeutic relationship that emerged helped Anna, toward the end of the first year of analysis, disclose an extremely important secret to me. Anna spoke in depth about her feelings of estrangement in Israel. I could easily identify with this, remembering my own feelings of uprootedness and vulnerability as a new immigrant. The reason that Anna gave for feeling so foreign was unexpected: 'I am not Jewish. I do not belong here,' she said. 'Nobody knows about this; it is a secret'. I was very surprised indeed. If there is a typical Jewish appearance, Anna had it. It fleetingly occurred to me that her brown hair and beautiful brown eyes would have definitely endangered her life during the Holocaust.

The story that followed revealed that Anna and her husband had had a considerable struggle to get out of Romania. At that time, because the privilege of leaving Romania was given only to Jews, she and her husband had searched for a Jewish connection. Anna's husband discovered that his mother's first husband was Jewish. This fact, in addition to a large bribe paid to Romanian officials, enabled the couple to obtain the false papers necessary for being considered Jewish, thus enabling them to immigrate to Israel.

My gut reaction to Anna's story was the wish to console her. 'Who cares whether you are Jewish or not?' I wanted to say to her. However, aware that my impulse to deny Anna's feelings of being a stranger probably stemmed from my own painful memories as a child in Romania, I remained quiet.

My first memory evoked by Anna's story was that of the complicated world of a Jewish child from a rabbinic family growing up with a Christian Adventist nanny, who faithfully took me to Adventist services on Friday afternoons (of course, without my parents' knowledge!). I remember loving Jesus and the beautiful pictures and sculptures of him. How great was my frustration when I discovered that, being Jewish, Jesus was not our God! Also, growing up among Christian Orthodox children I learned that we, the Jewish people, were accused of having killed Jesus and were therefore damned forever. My Hebrew name made the fact that I was Jewish, and thus a foreigner, obvious to everyone.

On the other hand, I remembered that coming to Israel, the country we had longed for, and living among Jewish people, did little to alleviate my feelings of being an outsider. In the new country, children looked and behaved differently; they spoke a language totally foreign to me. It took a long time for me to feel at home, and I never completely acquired the sense of belonging that I had so desired.

Based on my countertransference feelings, I asked Anna if she thought that her feelings of being a foreigner stemmed from immigrating to Israel. Anna reflected and said quietly, 'Actually, I have felt a stranger all my life'. Anna added that in her neighbourhood in Romania there were many German-speaking people as well as Jews, and as a result, she understood both German and Yiddish. 'I always admired the Jewish people and wanted to live among them. They are clever and witty,' she said, smiling.

What a strange world, I thought to myself. As a child I wanted to belong to the Christian majority, which I felt was all-powerful, and Anna wanted to belong to the Jewish minority, which she imagined was superior. This childhood experience that we both shared, a longing to belong to another nationality, had an impact on me as well as on the therapeutic relationship. I realised that, as children, we unconsciously longed for a happier, better-integrated family, and we projected the qualities of strength of body and mind onto each other's ethnic group. Based on my own realisation, I pointed out to Anna that she perhaps had always wished to have a happier family, and that she imagined this family to be Jewish.

Anna was able to accept this interpretation, which facilitated the further working through of the painful love-hate relationship that characterised her attitude toward her own family. We first elaborated upon the feelings that accompanied the loss of her parents. She recounted at length her mother's terrible suffering and death; her mother had died of brain cancer when Anna was 21. Anna and her older sister lived with their mother, who had devoted her life to the care of her daughters. Her parents divorced when Anna was around 12 years old. She witnessed many violent quarrels between her parents, and always felt that she had to protect her mother from her brutal father. She remembered the bitter day when her father left home and moved to the city. He was a well-known musician with many women friends. Her poor mother worked long hours as a cashier in a store and was barely able to support her children. Her dream was that her daughters would have an education and Anna, the brilliant medical student, fulfilled her mother's dream. Anna was very attached to her mother and did everything she could to make her happy.

When she was an adolescent, Anna occasionally visited her father. Anna liked him; he was very charming and seductive. He took her to concerts where he presented her as his young mistress and invited her to restaurants with his friends. After a while, her father became very depressed. He became an alcoholic and abandoned his work at the orchestra. Two years after her mother's death he was found dead in his apartment, probably as a result of alcohol and drugs.

During the year of her mother's illness, Anna took constant care of her. Though trying hard to study as well, she was unable to concentrate. Her mother died and Anna failed her final exams.

Anna left home after her mother's death and moved to the city. Her sister was already married with children. Anna felt completely abandoned and was unable to mourn her mother or, later, her father. She had an unhappy affair with a man she did not love, followed by an abortion. Anna was depressed, unable to continue her studies or find work.

In the midst of this chaotic, fragmented life, she regained control of her faculties and decided to re-register at the university to retake the courses she had failed. There, she met a young man, her future husband, who gave her much love and support. The relationship had parental aspects that Anna very much needed. She loved her husband, and they decided together to immigrate to Israel and build a new life.

Anna's maternal grandmother, who lived in Romania, died while Anna was in analysis. This event put Anna in touch with a great deal of grief and pain. Working through this powerful outburst of mourning in analysis made Anna aware that she had never actually mourned her parents. Anna expressed a wish to visit her parents' graves, as well as that of her grandmother to whom she had been very attached. I felt that Anna had to return to her country of origin in order to complete her work of mourning. She had to mourn her lost loved ones as well as the parts of her own self that had remained there. Anna longed to see the colour of the trees, the familiar streets and houses and her childhood home. She also wanted to visit her sister and family, to bring them presents from Israel and to bring back some of her personal belongings that she had left behind. In analysis, I felt that Anna was asking me to give her the courage and support to undertake the visit.

When Anna returned to analysis three weeks later, after her visit, she looked different. The depression that had accompanied her before was gone, and it was replaced by a statement of loss and pain. During this period, we were able to work through her love and longing for her mother, as well as her anger at being abandoned by her when she was so young and helpless. We discovered that behind the bitterness toward her abandoning father were feelings of pity and sorrow, as well as love and admiration.

Much psychic work was needed for the completion of Anna's work of mourning. The elaboration on the visit to her parents' graves, its emotional meaning, and the separation from her parents preoccupied us for an entire year. At the end of this year, Anna came to her session smiling and asked me if I was ready for a surprise. Radiant with happiness, she broke the good news: 'I am pregnant', she said, 'and it took me only one month'.

Anna was elated, and I rejoiced in her happiness. I accompanied Anna through her pregnancy, which included all of the normal anxieties and expectations of a young mother. Knowing that she would have a boy, she raised the question of circumcision. (Jewish males are circumcised at the age of eight days, this being considered a sign of the covenant between the God of Israel and his people.) In the end, she made her decision: 'I want my boy to be circumcised. He lives in this country, and he will be like everyone else'. Her husband was of the same opinion.

When her analysis ended some months later, Anna promised to come back and visit me. She indeed came to see me two years later with a most adorable toddler. She had completed her internship, had begun working as a psychiatrist, and the family's economic situation had improved. She had recently heard from some colleagues that I was planning to go to Bucharest for work and she was very excited about that. 'I would very much like to go with you, to take you around, to help you there', she said. 'You helped me go back and find myself. You gave me a lot and I would have liked to reciprocate', she added in her beautiful, elegant Romanian.

In the autumn of that year, 36 years after leaving the country, I returned to Romania in a professional capacity. A colleague met me at the airport and, at my request, we immediately set out to find my childhood home. We reached my old neighbourhood that was so familiar to me, and I easily found my way around. I looked at the houses, churches, and streets that were imprinted upon my memory and walked about as if in a dream.

When I arrived at the square where my parents' house was supposed to be, I was struck by the strange sight that unfolded before my eyes: The left-hand side of the square looked the same as I remembered it, but the right-hand side, where our house once stood, had changed completely. Stunned, I stood in front of the square, asking myself over and over again, 'But where is the house? Where is it?'. My colleague, who had already warned me that parts of Bucharest had completely disappeared during the rule of Nicolae Ceausescu, patiently explained to me what I already knew. Ceausescu, the former dictator of Romania, had destroyed entire neighbourhoods; beautiful historical buildings and churches that had given the city its very special character had been torn down indiscriminately. In their place, architectural monsters had been erected, their ugly grandiosity reminiscent of the Fascist era, as well as of Ceausescu's megalomaniacal wishes, ruthlessness, and oppression.

The same traumatic experience confronted me when I attempted to find my grandparents' house. The house, which had also served as a synagogue in the Jewish community and in which I had lived until the age of four, held some of my earliest memories. I still remembered the sun shining through the leaves of the tree in the big yard where I played. I also remembered the Torah scroll in the synagogue, as well as my grandmother's big kitchen where, as a young child, I enjoyed cooking with her. This house had been the container of feelings of warmth and love, and my memories of it had served as a source of strength and courage during difficult moments of my life.

Staring at the new surroundings for some time, I realised that both my parents' and grandparents' houses had vanished into thin air. Feelings of anger overwhelmed me. After working them through, they gave way to feelings of sorrow. I felt as if the houses were parts of myself that were irretrievably lost. I became aware that, although I had done much work of mourning throughout my life, it was far from complete. Working through my mourning, I thought often of Anna, my Romanian patient. I realised the impact that the treatment had had on both of us. Not only had I helped Anna in the search for herself but, by assisting her on her journey back to her homeland, I myself was better prepared for the visit back to my birthplace. Thus, Anna's wish to accompany me on my journey back to my country of birth was realised, at least in fantasy.

As the Romanian-born philosopher and essayist, E.M. Cioran wrote in 1960: 'I would give all the landscapes of the world for that of my childhood. I must add, though, that if I make a paradise out of it, only the tricks of infirmity of memory can be held responsible' (Cioran 1960, p. 12; quoted in Amati-Mehler, Argentieri and Canestri, 1993 and in S. Akhtar, 1999, p. 89).

Those who stayed behind – an emigrant society

In January 2001, my book *The Cry of Mute Children,* which deals with the understanding and treatment of second-generation Holocaust survivors, appeared in Romanian, published by Editura Trei (Kogan, 1995). The book's main themes are, first, the transmission of trauma from one generation to another and, second, the creation of hope and the reconstruction of the self-image. I feel that these two themes are relevant to Romanian society and to anyone whose life has been touched by the reality of war, violence, and trauma. The Romanian people suffered the trauma of living under a dictatorship that ruled by terror and violence. Not only did they live lives of sheer misery, but they had also been humiliated and infantilised. In my encounters with local Romanians, I have seen a lack of self-assurance, a derogatory attitude toward themselves and a lack of belief in their ability to create a better future. The many years of oppression and terror had left a deep imprint on their psychic make-up.

Over the past few years I have taken an active part in the establishment of the Psychotherapy Centre for the Treatment of the Child and Adolescent in Bucharest, the first of its kind in Romania. Here is how this centre came into being: on one of my visits to Romania in a professional capacity, to work with Romanian therapists, I was met at the airport by a colleague, Vera Sandor. It was December, the trees were covered with a heavy blanket of snow, and there was a thin layer of ice on the ground, which I was told was very slippery and dangerous. During our ride from the airport, I was deep in thought, looking at the beautiful patterns that the snowflakes created on the windscreen, patterns that reminded me of scenes from my childhood. At a traffic light, I saw a small dark figure banging on the window. Startled, I asked Vera, 'What is that?' 'A street child,' she replied calmly. Then she went on to explain about the life of street children, which I was familiar with only from Western literature on Romania. The traffic light changed, and we drove off. However, the face of that little child continued to haunt me for a long time.

It was during this visit that Vera talked about her dream of setting up the Psychotherapy Centre for the Treatment of the Child and Adolescent in Romania. 'There are houses for street children, but they usually run away from them. We should find better ways to deal with that, but it is also vital that we prevent others from becoming street children. As you know, there are lots of families in Romania with problematic children who are not on the streets, and these children have no place to turn for help,' she said. This is very true, I thought, and I wondered what was happening to those children who did have families, food, and clothing, but who were also suffering from psychic problems. Their future is grim, and they could end up becoming thieves, criminals, psychotics, or drug addicts. Shouldn't we use our knowledge and experience to avoid such catastrophes that could affect their lives and the shape of an entire society?

Leaving Romania for Hamburg to work with my colleague and friend Professor Peter Riedesser, I shared with him the dream of setting up such a centre in Bucharest. Peter, a man of vision, enthusiastically became part of this enterprise.

I will not go into the details of the long journey we both made in order to realise this dream. Suffice it to say that after the many difficulties and disappointments that we encountered along the way, there were people who had faith in our work and goals, and who helped us set up the centre in Bucharest.

During my many subsequent visits to Romania, I supervised the work of the staff as well as the centre's activities and goals and I learned how Romanian society had reacted to the abrupt change from a totalitarian Communist regime to a Western lifestyle. Discussions with friends, colleagues and students showed me that the general feelings toward the totalitarian regime were disappointment, hatred and impotence. In spite of this, the Romanian people still felt some yearning for the past. This phenomenon is frequently found in many countries that become westernised. What is unique about Romanian society is that it suffers from a state of unresolved mourning for a dictator who they themselves eliminated. This pathological mourning for old values and for the image of the lost dictator made it more difficult for Romanian society to integrate the new attitudes and values of the new era.

Entering a new era, Romanians were first forced to revaluate old principles and adapt to different values. They could envision promising opportunities, but these were accompanied by alien, burdensome requirements. They had to abruptly exchange the rituals and teachings of a familiar culture for a new, unfamiliar situation (Kahn, 1997).

In addition, the totalitarian Communist regime had stifled initiative for private enterprise as well as the motivation needed to achieve an improved work ethic and a higher standard of living. The state had provided a secure, albeit very low salary for the people, independent of the quality of their work. There was equality in this situation, since a life of deprivation was almost everyone's fate. Basic needs, such as health and education, were taken care of by the state. This infantilised the population, making them unable to take responsibility for their own lives.

The new post-Communist era also created turmoil in peoples' lives. Despite the promise of freedom and opportunity, the immediate reality required skills that had not been developed for a long time and a motivation to work, to which they were unaccustomed. The Romanian people also experienced narcissistic hurt when comparing their lives to life in the West and in particular to that of the other westernised countries of Eastern Europe; this was also accompanied by feelings of shame and humiliation. In comparison with the West, their own living quarters and attire took on a shabbiness that they regarded with the embarrassment of the newly poor. In the most part, they still considered themselves incapable of coping in a competitive economy; they were embarrassed by their inexperience in carrying out the complex practices fundamental to the democratic process.

As a result of these changes, the Romanian people came to feel the humiliation of the breadwinner's vocational worthlessness in the workplace and resultant loss of status within the family. The purchasing power of their savings and their modest pensions became insignificant. From my encounters with the group that initiated the centre, I learned that Romanian society looked upon the West with awe and suspicion. When I told his group about the efforts made in the West to help them construct the centre, they asked fearfully, 'Why do they want to do this for us?'. I then realised that one of my first roles would be to serve as a bridge to the West, one that would allow the people to build a future relationship of trust.

Discussion

In my discussion, I first focus on the impact that emigration had on the sense of identity and the mourning process of the patient described in the first part of this chapter. I then briefly relate this process to mourning process on a social level.

The capacity to maintain a sense of consolidated identity (sameness amid change) was first noted by Erikson (1950, 1956). More recently, Stern (1985), through his recent concept of 'self-history' (that is, a sense of continuation with one's subjective past), refers to this same capacity. In trying to clarify the concept of identity, Akhtar (1999) has noted that individuals with a solid identity retain genuine ties with their past while comfortably locating themselves in their current reality.

The drastic alteration of external reality resulting from migration from one country to another produces a profound psychic flux and has an impact on an individual's identity. Loss of familiar landscape, music, food, language, and customs mobilises pain and mourning (Grinberg and Grinberg, 1989). Such mourning and 'culture-shock' (Garza-Guerrero, 1974) cause a destabilisation of identity, and it takes considerable time and intrapsychic work to settle and restabilise itself. However, in instances where the pre-emigration character structure is problematic, where the intrapsychic separateness did not exist before emigration, the consolidation of identity may be hindered all the more.

In the case of Anna, the patient came to treatment with conflicts that had already afflicted her sense of identity. As a child, her ethnic or national self-representation was laden with shame and she idealised the Jewish identity. When she became an immigrant in Israel, she felt as vulnerable as a child and her devaluation of her country of origin as well as of her own self was reinforced. Much psychic work was needed to change this devaluating attitude, which stemmed from early traumatic experiences as well as from her incomplete work of mourning.

Anna suffered not only the loss of her mother and father; by emigrating, she also lost the support she had drawn from the familiar climate and landscape, unconsciously perceived as the extension of the mother. Her wish to return for a visit to her native land, which emerged in analysis, was very much linked to her longing for lost primary objects as well as the need to give them up and build a life of her own. Revisiting her parents' graves helped her achieve this aim and held great psychic significance for her (Akhtar and Smolar, 1998). By taking gifts to relatives left behind and by bringing some of her personal belongings back with her to her new home, Anna made the first attempts at separation, like a toddler in the rapprochement phase.

Before she began analysis, the patient had not yet given up primary objects or familiar places through the work of mourning, nor assimilated them in the ego through identification. This resulted in a temporal 'fracture of the psyche' (Akhtar, 1999). One of the aims of her analysis was to help her put together the different fragments of her psyche, as well as the various 'pieces of her life' (Pfeiffer, 1974). The 'holding relationship' (Kogan, 1995, 1996, 1998, 2000, 2002) in analysis helped her mobilise forces and go back and face the 'mental pain' (Freud, 1926) incurred in the acknowledgement of her losses. This dynamic shift helped Anna continue her work of mourning in analysis.

The great disparities between their lives before and after the fall of Communism as well as the abruptness of the change, left people yearning for what they had left behind. In this new situation, which had its uncomfortable and painful aspects, many felt nostalgic for past Communist ideals and even dared to secretly express a longing for the former dictator. The corruption, betrayal and terrorisation by the former Communist government were partially experienced as an idealised parent who had been exposed as corrupt or inhuman. The experience of loss of the old culture intensified, accompanied by anxiety, hostility and a 'sense of discontinuity of identity' (Garza-Guerrero, 1974). The destruction of former identifications, as well as the loss of the accustomed life, brought with it depression and feelings of loneliness. The prolonged despair was due in great part to the difficulty of working through processes of mourning.

Freud defined mourning as 'the reaction to the loss of a loved person, or to the loss of some abstraction which has taken the place of one, such as one's country, liberty, an ideal and so on' (Freud, 1917, p. 243). For the individual, mourning is an obligatory psychobiological process. In normal situations, if someone dies, we have to do much work to let that person die psychologically. Without going through the work of mourning, we cannot genuinely accept the reality that something is lost. And if the lost person is needed for our psychological well-being, or if he or she forms a part of our own ego-ideal (Joffe and Sandler, 1965; Sandler, Holder, and Meers 1987), we may slip into a state of pathological mourning.

Romanian society was for a long time marked and characterised by unresolved mourning for their dreadful leader, Nicolae Ceausescu. Volkan (1998) convincingly bases his analysis of the relationship between Romanians and their dictator on Freud's (1913) psychoanalytic understanding of primitive man. Volkan claims that although the Romanians executed Ceausescu, they allowed him to live on in many ways – most importantly, through the actions and policies that followed his death. Their pathological mourning was expressed through the fact that they could not eliminate the image of the leader (the father figure) but instead kept it alive through hatred as well as nostalgia.

Romanians rejoiced over the removal of Ceausescu but after the initial excitement, most felt that little had changed. Many considered the National Salvation Front (NSF) merely an anti-Ceausescu faction within the Romanian Communist Party and regarded the new regime simply as a replacement of one group of Communists with another.

The Romanian people never fully realised that although the reign of Nicolae Ceausescu had ended, his 'sons' had not only 'murdered' him but also kept him alive. Having ruled the Romanian people for two decades, Ceausescu had become a part of them. With his death, a part of each Romanian had also died (Grinberg, 1964), but the shame of being associated with him and their hidden guilt for 'killing' him had to be denied.

However, through their identification with the dictator they were also keeping him alive.

In June 1990, nationalists launched a weekly publication called *Romania Mare* [Great Romania], a reference to the centuries-old, traditional rallying cry of Romanian nationalists before Ceausescu's rise to power. The paper, which developed the largest circulation of any Romanian weekly newspaper, succeeded in keeping Ceausescu 'alive' through an undisguised nostalgia for his regime. In 2000, the head of this weekly publication, Corneliu Vadim Tudor, became the head of the largest opposition party to the new government, almost endangering its existence. The party received a great number of votes, promising to 'purify' Romania of the gypsy population, the Hungarian minority, and the Mafia, while emphasising Romanian nationalism. Despite the fact that the NSF was re-elected, a rejection of democracy by many Romanians and a longing for the past dictatorship became quite obvious. By identifying with the aggressor, the Romanians had internalised the image of the dreaded leader and made it part of themselves (Volkan, 1998).

As in the case of my patient and myself, the efforts and willingness of my Romanian colleagues to accompany me on my journey back to my childhood may perhaps be viewed as an expression of their own need to search for their past in order to complete their own work of mourning.

Note

1. This chapter was previously published in Ilany Kogan (2007), *The Struggle against Mourning* (Chapter 4). Plymouth: Jason Aronson/Lanham, MD: Rowman and Littlefield and is reprinted here with the kind permission of the author and the publishers. Minor spelling changes have been made by the editors to comply with British spelling in this book.

References

Akhtar, S. (1999). *Immigration and Identity: Turmoil, Treatment and Transformation*. Northvale, NJ: Jason Aronson.

Akhtar, S., and Smolar, A. (1998). Visiting the father's grave. *Psychoanalytic Quarterly 67*(3), 474–83.

Amati-Mehler, J., Argentieri, S., and Canestri, J. (1993). *The Babel of the Unconscious: Mother Tongue and Foreign Languages in the Psychoanalytic Dimension*, trans. J. Whitelaw-Cucco. Madison, CT: International Universities Press.

Anzieu, D. (1976). L'enveloppe sonore du Soi. *Nouvelle Revue de Psychanalyse*, *13*, 161–79.

Cioran, E.M. (1960). *History and Utopia*, trans. by R. Howard (2015). New York: Arcade Publishing.

Erikson, E.H. ([1950]1959). Growth and crises of the healthy personality. In *Identity and the Life Cycle* (pp. 50–100). New York: International University Press.

Erikson, E.H. (1956). The problem of ego identity. *Journal of the American Psychoanalytic Association*, *4*(1), 56–121.

Freud, S. (1913). Totem and Taboo. *Standard Edition, Vol. XIII* (pp. 1–162). London: Hogarth Press.

Freud, S. (1917). Mourning and Melancholia. *Standard Edition, Vol. XIV* (pp. 237–59). London: Hogarth Press.

Freud, S. (1926). Inhibitions, Symptoms and Anxiety. *Standard Edition, Vol. XX* (pp. 77–174). London: Hogarth Press.

Garza-Guerrero, A.C. (1974). Culture shock: its mourning and the vicissitudes of identity. *Journal of the American Psychoanalytic Association, 22*(2), 408–29.

Grinberg, L. (1964). Two kinds of guilt: their relations with normal and pathological aspects of mourning. *International Journal of Psychoanalysis, 45*, 366–71.

Grinberg, L., and R. Grinberg, S. (1989). *Psychoanalytic Perspectives on Migration and Exile*, trans. by N. Festinger. New Haven, CT and London: Yale University Press. Originally published as *Psicoanálisis de la migración y del exilio*. Madrid: Alianza, 1984 (Editorial).

Joffe, W.G., and Sandler, J. ([1965]1987). Pain, Depression and Individuation. In J. Sandler. (ed.), *From Safety to Superego*. London: Karnac.

Kahn, C. (1997). Emigration Without Leaving Home. In P.H. Elovitz and C. Kahn (eds), *Immigrant Experiences: Personal Narrative and Psychological Analysis*. Madison, Teaneck: Farleigh Dickinson University Press.

Kogan, I. (1995). *The Cry of Mute Children: A Psychoanalytic Perspective of the Second Generation of the Holocaust*. London and New York: Free Association Books.

Kogan, I. (1996). Die Suche nach Geschichte in den Analysen der Nachkommen von Holocaust-Überlebenden: Rekonstruktion des 'seelischen Lochs'. In H. Weiss and H. Lang (eds), *Psychoanalyse Heute Und Vor 70 Jahren*. Tubingen: edition diskord, pp. 201–308. Also in: M. Endres and G. Biermann (eds), *Traumatisierung in Kindheit and Jugend* (pp. 83–98). Munich and Basel: Ernst Reinhardt Verlag, 1998.

Kogan, I. (1998). The Black Hole of Dread: The Psychic Reality of Children of Holocaust Survivors. In J.H. Berke, S. Pierides, A. Sobbaddini and S. Schneider (eds) *Even Paranoids Have Enemies: New Perspectives on Paranoia and Persecution* (pp. 47–59). London and New York: Routledge.

Kogan, I. (2000). Breaking the cycle of trauma: from the individual to society. *Mind and Human Interaction, 11*, 2–10.

Kogan, I. (2002). 'Enactment' in lives and treatment of Holocaust survivors' offspring. *Psychoanalytic Quarterly, 71*(2), 251–73.

Kogan, I. (2007). *The Struggle against Mourning*. Plymouth: Jason Aronson and Lanham, MD: Rowman and Littlefield.

Pfeiffer, E. (1974). Borderline states. *Disorders of the Nervous System, 35*, 212–19.

Sandler, J., Holder, A., and Meers, D. (1987). Ego-ideal and ideal self. In J. Sandler (ed.) *From Safety to Superego* (pp. 73–90). London: Karnac.

Stein, J., and Urdang, L. (eds) (1968). *The Random House Dictionary of the English Language*. New York: Random House.

Stern, D. (1985). *The Interpersonal World of the Infant*. New York: Basic Books.

Volkan, V. (1998). Totem and Taboo in Romania: The Internalization of a 'Dead' Leader and Re-stabilization of an Ethnic Tent. In *Blood Lines: From Ethnic Pride to Ethnic Terrorism*. (pp. 181–202). Boulder: Westview Press.

Zac de Filc, S. (1992). Psychic change in the analyst. *International Journal of Psychoanalysis, 73*(Pt 2), 323–9.

Chapter 5

Tolerance for non-understanding: understanding and its limits – the confusion of tongues[1,2]

Nadja Gogolin

Babel

> Now the whole earth had one language and the same words. And as the people migrated from the east, they found a plain in the land of Shinar and settled there. And they said one to another, 'Come, let us make bricks, and burn them thoroughly'. And they had brick for stone, and bitumen for mortar. Then they said, 'Come, let us build ourselves a city and a tower with its top in the heavens, and let us make us a name for ourselves, lest we be dispersed over the face of the whole earth.' And the Lord came down to see the city and the tower, which the children of man had built. And the Lord said, 'Behold, they are one people, and they have one language, and this is only the beginning of what they will do. And nothing that they propose to do will now be impossible for them. Come, let us go down, and confuse their language, so that they may not understand one another's speech.' So the Lord dispersed them from there over the face of the earth, and they left off building the city. Therefore its name was called Babel, because the Lord confused the language of all the earth. And from there, the Lord dispersed them over the face of all the earth.
>
> Genesis 11:1–9.

Babel still stands for 'confounding' or 'confusion' today. Confusion, lack of understanding and not feeling understood are fundamental experiences in psychotherapy. In contrast to that experience, however, is the opposite wish – even the believed phantasy – of a complete and total understanding. In this chapter, I set out to describe how this phantasy and the inevitable disappointment when confronted with the limits of reality, shapes the experience of migrant patients in Berlin who are treated with group analysis in their English mother tongue.

When we try to understand a person, we will always be confronted with the limits of our capacity to understand since understanding, insight and closeness are always relative and limited. It is one of the main tasks of psychotherapy to recognise these limitations of reality, to help our patients to accept it and to live with it. In *The Babel of the Unconscious* (1993), Amati-Mehler, Argentieri and Canestri discuss how the longing for a total understanding came about using the biblical picture of the pre-Babel World: 'Now the whole earth had one language and the same words'. They show us how the myth of a single language brings to life this longing for unlimited mutual understanding, although it does not exist outside of the myth itself. But within the myth, the 'one language' and 'one speech' which suggests limitless understanding, are presented as if they actually existed in reality – in fact, in prehistoric times. Psychoanalysis understands this prehistoric picture in terms of an unconscious picture of the mind, a phantasy and yearning for something that, although it is an unattainable ideal, is alive in everyone's phantasy as something that acts as a memory.

According to Amati-Mehler, Argentieri and Canestri, there is also a 'regressive' aspect in the myth because the prehistoric state of 'one language' fulfils also the longing for an 'eternal homecoming'. In psychoanalytic terms this is understood as a wish for the experience of merging. The 'progressive' aspect, on the other hand, is the experience of difference, separateness and sacrifice: 'The Lord dispersed them' and 'confused the languages'. From a psychoanalytic point of view, this expresses the other pole of the existential dilemma, the pole of limitation and finiteness, sacrifice and the impossibility of having everything or being everything.

In addition to the archaic state of the shared language with its associated possibility of unlimited understanding and the unhappy final state of the confusion of tongues, the myth also includes a deed and a subsequent punishment: banishment and exile. The deed is the building of the tower 'with its top in the heaven' and the punishment is the confusion of language and the subsequent shattering of the plan to build the tower. Psychoanalytically, this can be read as a metaphor to express the painful process of development. In order to develop, we have to renounce omnipotence phantasy and accept differentiation and the limitations that come with it, also the limits of understanding. Nevertheless, we never stop yearning for total understanding and we continue to try to find it.

In psychotherapy, the attempt to arrive at an understanding is made on the level of language. Language is our medium. We may and must do all we can to ensure that as good an understanding as possible is achieved. And we are also only able to 'touch' with words. I am a German psychoanalyst working with patients whose mother tongue, English, is different from mine. I need to be particularly aware of the potential, even probable limits to my understanding, not only in general, but also in relation to the language difference. At the same time, the wish for limitless understanding is ubiquitous, also in those whose mother tongue is different and who come to me in need of therapy. I can describe the people with whom I embark on a therapeutic process in their native language in terms of the internal aspects of their mind or in terms of outer aspects of their external world. There is, however, no clear dividing line between the two. In the tension between understanding and non-understanding, I consider it important to stay within an area midway between understanding and non-understanding which I find tolerable.

The mother tongue of the patients with whom I declare myself willing to work is, though not mine, familiar to me. Likewise, the culture of the patients is different from mine, but relatively familiar to me. One might refer to it as 'Western Culture'. The patients in my groups come from the UK, US, Ireland, Canada and Australia. I feel that I am able to understand this culture, within my own limits, and that there is more that connects us than separates us. They are living here in Germany in voluntary exile, that is, forced by internal circumstances, but not by external ones. In his article, *The foreign citizen as a mass phenomenon* (Abel, 2011), Thomas Abel has written about different groups of immigrants who seek psychotherapy in Germany. According to his classification, my patients are people whose reasons for immigrating were internal. They differ from those who come to Germany having fled or been expelled from their home countries, or who have needed to leave for material reasons. The difference is that those in voluntary exile can decide to return. They may be equally traumatised and often are, but their trauma is a kind of relationship trauma, such as we might also encounter in German patients.

According to Abel, people who migrate for internal reasons usually come from countries that are similar to ours in terms of culture, economic system and religion. Psychotherapy is usually expensive in the English-speaking home countries of my patients. Patients are often well-informed concerning the psychotherapeutic services available to them in the German health system. In my experience, these patients often appreciate these services far more than German patients. Another reason for choosing Germany as their country of voluntary exile can sometimes be found in patients of Jewish origin who come in search of their family history. The descendants of Jewish families who had been forced to emigrate or who fell victim to the Holocaust, have surnames that betray their German background. They may know of grandmothers, or of a whole (often gruelling) history – or they may know nothing of their family history in Germany and bring with them instead a sense of something being missing which acts as a mission or an unspoken commission that guides their search here, a search that is initially often undefined.

I work with patients who have usually had to leave their home countries for internal reasons. While most of these patients have indeed experienced trauma, this is usually the same kind of attachment trauma that we encounter in German patients. As Thomas Abel has also described in the paper mentioned above, the migration from the former German Democratic Republic to a unified Germany which I also experienced, took place without my having moved an inch. It took place because the Wall between East and West Germany came down in 1989. Perhaps this experience of migration makes it easier for me to understand the loss of one's linguistic and cultural sphere. That is something which I share with my patients, the experience of a change that I welcomed and valued, and an exile that was voluntary, but nevertheless a traumatic experience to be taken seriously.

In my opinion, these patients, whom I treat in a group therapy setting, can have an effective therapeutic experience in Germany precisely because it is a foreign country to them and at the same time, they can use (and may in fact need to use) their mother tongue. They can make use of the fact that they are in exile and as exiles they benefit in particular from the group setting. Group psychotherapy offers a containing space and an intermediate area of experience after traumatic experiences of non-understanding in childhood as well as the ruptures in understanding involved in migration. If we accept that there are internal reasons for migration, we must also assume that the wish to be heard and understood has already been thwarted earlier in life. If it is an inner sense of disappointment in the internal home within the self which leads to the decision to set out to find a new home, then the phantasy of total understanding will often be carried over into the new country. A disappointing reality is left behind in order to search for a 'better' one elsewhere.

When the conditions into which a child is born do not provide it with that which it needs to develop sufficient trust in its human environment, it will continue to mistrust closeness and intimacy throughout life. If the disappointment and hurt come from those persons on which the child is dependent for protection and comfort, the child is especially likely to become mistrustful, not only towards those to whom he is close, but of closeness and intimacy as such.

Leaving one's home country also involves a number of potentially traumatic experiences, most notably loss, that is, the loss of a containing environment, both in its animate and inanimate aspects. Depending on each person's individual personality and previous life experiences, this will have more or less severe ramifications.

Winnicott (see also Grinberg and Grinberg, 1989, p. 14) has described the importance of 'transitional phenomena' in the 'intermediate area of experience' or the 'potential space' between the individual and the environment for the development of a 'true', that is, 'creative' self. Throughout life, the 'cultural inheritance' – as an extension of each person's 'potential space' – between an individual and his environment helps a person to feel the continuity of his or her existence:

> It is useful then, to think of a third area of human living, one neither inside the individual nor outside in the world of shared reality. This intermediate living can be thought of as occupying a potential space,

> negating the idea of space and separation between the baby and the mother, and all developments derived from this phenomenon.
>
> (Winnicott, 1971, p. 110)

> There is a direct development from transitional phenomena to playing, and from playing to shared playing, and from this to cultural experiences ... Playing implies trust, and belongs to the potential space between (what was at first) baby and mother-figure, with the baby in a state of near-absolute dependence, and the mother-figure's adaptive function taken for granted by the baby.
>
> (Winnicott, pp. 51–2)

> The place where cultural experience is located is in the *potential space* between the individual and the environment (originally the object). The same can be said of playing. Cultural experience begins with creative living first manifested in play.
>
> (Winnicott, p. 100)

But when crisis and rupture occur, as it may in migration, cultural inheritance cannot provide the necessary containment. A containing and intermediate area of experience might then become necessary in which the crisis can be worked through in relative safety. Psychotherapy offers that area of relative safety, and the analytic group is a specific variety of that safe space, offering the potential space in the native language of its members. In this it is similar to the developmental needs of a child. When a child experiences a prolonged absence from his mother, he loses the capacity to symbolise. The capacity for playing and exploration is also compromised and the child has to revert to more primitive defence mechanisms. In the same way, a deprived immigrant also suffers from a diminished capacity for creativity and cultural experience. To regain her or his abilities, the immigrant has to work through and overcome the deprivation. Group therapy can offer a helpful space in which the experience of loss and deprivation can first be shared and then acknowledged in order to overcome the resentful states of mind that are often held onto for defensive reasons with feelings of having been wronged, deprived and victimised.

Among the many reasons people might have for leaving their home country, trying to get away from an unbearable inner conflict or developmental task, and the connected wish to change countries in order not to change the inner conflict is the reason that most frequently leads to the need for psychotherapeutic treatment in the new environment. There are two factors that come together in such cases: The insecure attachment that developed in early childhood had already compromised the ability to address and resolve their conflicts in their country of origin. By leaving their home country, they hope to leave these conflicts behind. But the unresolved issues manifest themselves again in their diminished capacity to integrate into the new environment. Thus the 'not good enough' inner reality is replicated in the external 'not good enough' reality in their new home. According to attachment theory, all of us remain dependent on attachment figures to whom we can turn in times of need and anxiety throughout our lives. Early attachment trauma impairs or destroys the capacity to turn trustingly to others because the fear of a repetition of the old traumatic experience is too threatening.

Migration can reactivate this early experience. To lose one's home country, language, familiar people and skills is in itself traumatic. However, migrants also lose the very people to whom they could have turned in their distress (see Holmes, 2010, p. 136). The migration itself can be understood in terms of a series of micro-traumas that can result in a crisis. The original deficits are thus repeated: the lack of a containing object or environment or a potential space that would enable the individual to work through the pain of loss and the overwhelming, unbearable affects. Moreover, in our contemporary, globalised world we are easily tempted to escape from (intra-psychic) situations that appear insoluble, by fleeing geographically. As a result of this development, there is a risk that moving and travelling will be used defensively in the service of avoiding conflicts and in order to sustain an idealised inner and outer illusory world (White, 2011).

If there is no internal object that enables us to stay and endure or work through conflicts, then the stress and conflicts involved in the process of escaping by relocating will evoke the latent (primitive) defence of splitting that we typically encounter in our patients. Such patients have often created a split between their country of origin, which is initially hated, and the new country, which is yearned for and idealised. This idealisation is often followed by a disappointment, since idealisations are always followed by disappointment. We then observe a shift towards the opposite pole: Memories of the old country are idealised while the new country is perceived as disappointing, excluding and rejecting. This is repeated in the therapeutic relationship. Typically, after a certain period of treatment, the patient comes to feel disappointed in the therapist whom they had initially idealised as a saviour. The patient now experiences the therapist as withholding and inadequate, 'a mere human being' after all. If this – at that moment hurtful – perception of reality is seen to be an unalterable fact, then there is a risk that the patient will use travelling and feeling foreign in a foreign environment as a 'psychic retreat' (Steiner, 1993). The sadness and loss of the home country are denied. The fact that they have always felt 'foreign' even when they were 'at home', as well as the fact that this was one of their reasons for leaving in the first place, all of this then falls prey to denial. The external foreignness justifies the feeling of inner foreignness and the 'enemy' continues to be experienced as outside the self. In this, psychodynamic group therapy can be particularly helpful. Mathias Hirsch writes:

> The trauma destroys the capacity to symbolise, and also the ability to relate to other people. It splits off affects and impedes all access to them. Nowhere does one have such a good opportunity to experience what [and I would add 'that'] other people think about oneself and to express one's thoughts as in a psychoanalytic group. This is the place where the affects (which may initially be felt and expressed by someone else – a resonance phenomenon) can be regained, and also the place where trust in relationships with other people can grow, since in the group there is tolerance and a kind of non-moralistic ethics which demands only one thing: authenticity, that is, that one be true to oneself and not deceive oneself or the others, but embark on the quest for one's true identity (or at least not the victim identity of the traumatised) with the help of the other members of the group.
>
> (Hirsch, 2008, p. 823[3])

The group functions as a container where unconnected pieces of identity can be bound together and slowly integrated into a whole identity – much like a skin or the arms which hold the (psychic) parts of the infant together before the capacity for self-containment has been taken in.

All of the participants of the group share the experience of being 'in one boat'. They also share the opportunity to process the original split – the common enemy is Germany. The fact that all participants speak in their mother tongue in this group can also lead to unusual power relations. It is an unusual situation that they all speak English better than I do, even though I am fluent in English. Given that in therapy the imbalance of power is an often overlooked difficulty, this allows for a kind of 'empowerment' on the part of the group. Unlike in individual therapy, the group participants have the opportunity to perceive the similarities in their issues. Initially, this might lead to the group being misunderstood as a place that is all-good and conflict-free: 'At last I am among people who understand me and my problems with the world'. Then – fortunately always – the group becomes more like the real world and conflict occurs. It also contains people who are difficult to get on with and by whom one feels misunderstood, rejected, hated or ignored. And from this point on, the work can begin.

Clinical illustration

Jill is the mother of a daughter she has with a German husband who had persuaded her to come and stay in Germany. She met him when she was travelling through Europe – already conscious of her urge to travel, yet not to stay in one place for very long. Jill had spent her childhood years having to move back and forth between her mother's house on the Canadian border and her father's home town which was literally on the opposite side of the United States. Jill's mother had left when Jill was two years old. When she got back in touch a year after she had left, Jill no longer knew who the woman on the other end of the phone line even was. The arrangement to spend a year with each parent over the next ten years had left her deeply scarred. She could not develop any kind of trust in stability, in anything being reliable over time. When we met, she proudly told me that she could pack up and leave everything behind within five days. She had done it many times and had perfected the skill to form no deep attachment to anything or anybody.

The reason she came to therapy was the breakdown of her marriage. Given her history of losses, I offered Jill a place in the group. I was hoping for a fresh start for her in the country, which at this point in time held little to offer for her. She was bound to stay for the time being because her daughter wasn't ready to leave the country where her father lived. Her daughter was also the only person to whom Jill was attached. In the course of the months that we worked through Jill's recent and past experiences, she seemed to develop a basic trust in the group's reality, their interest and capacity to 'digest' her pain. Then – 'out of the blue' for all of us – it happened again. Jill had found a way to take her daughter with her and 'quit' – as she called it – Germany within 2 months. She was out of the group and the country faster than the group could grasp what was happening. The others had to work through the loss and the shock and yet they did not know what to make of it. At least the group was able to reflect back to Jill how she was repeating her early experience of sudden loss, of not being asked and being 'uprooted'.

Discussion

Understanding is a concept that is deeply embedded in language, words being spoken and listened to. In psychotherapy, where words are all we have, the language we use is very important. When we leave our country of origin and move to a country with another language, we also leave our mother tongue. We create a distance between language and everything that is (emotionally) encoded in this language. The words that stir us up (painfully) disappear from our daily lives. They can no longer affect us and no longer rekindle the old wounds. When patients speak several languages – and particularly when they have to learn a foreign language for the first time – what each language expresses and represents is a somewhat different symbolic world. 'Käse' is not cheese, 'Liebe' is not love, and 'Wut' and anger are not the same thing. Many of my patients speak German well enough to be able to do therapy in German, as a foreign language for them, of course. However, when the wounded part of the self exists in a language that is not spoken in the therapy, this can fuel a further splitting process in which something that is felt to be too painful to be touched is kept at arm's length. Thus, patients may also have (unconsciously) wished to migrate in order to lose their language.

I therefore believe that it is important for my patients to speak their mother tongue, even if it is not mine, to give them the opportunity to reach these wounded parts of themselves (also on a language level) and thus to learn to integrate the present and the past and the different parts of the self. While the loss of the ability to express ourselves through language is experienced as an affront and leaves us feeling helpless and excluded, it is – at the same time – a new beginning, and it is often defiantly countered with a (manic) defence against these very feelings of helplessness and exclusion. We then find individuals who manage to rapidly learn to speak the German language fluently, yet in the process, they leave themselves and their native language behind, as it were.

However, this type of rapid adaptation is also a reminder that (linguistic) exile is not only defensive, but also offers the hope of a creative new beginning. A new country is also a new start, a new try. Every action that replaces feeling and understanding stems from a compulsion to repeat an old traumatic experience (which is then repeated), but it also entails the hope for a better experience. If we did not understand that, psychotherapy, which aims for a better experience for the patient, would not be possible. Learning a new language entails an attempt to create better, less traumatic links and to leave the old ones behind. Expanding one's language skills and experience of the world lead to true psychological growth and an enhancement of the self. Our patients are searching for solutions; otherwise they would not embark on psychotherapy.

Internal and external boundaries

What appears in the myth of the Tower of Babel as a punishment – expulsion and exile which we also read as the end of an era of unbounded understanding – is our patients' (frequently self-chosen) reality. They experience an (internal) boundary, cross an (external) boundary and find themselves in a different country. From there they look and can (hopefully), with the help of therapy, see something that they could not have seen if they had not moved. They can discover their losses, their restrictions, their personal limitations, but also their potential. They need to have the experience of a boundary in order to be able to escape from the state of non-separation, in which they long for a state of merging and oneness that is free from tension and is 'all good' (but without an identity of their own). Through the experience of boundaries, they can begin to build up their own identities and achieve separateness. This allows them to grow, mourn, acknowledge reality and become adults in the broadest sense of the word. 'Without a boundary that reveals the moment where separation and renunciation of what is identical, undifferentiated and "lawless" there is no knowledge' (Amati-Mehler, Argentieri and Canestri, 1993, p. 18).

I believe that the patients whom I treat – often in groups – can have this experience outside of their home countries – that they have crossed an external boundary because they have come up against an internal boundary. In the psychoanalytic group they can – this is the hope – see something that they were unable to 'see' from the other side of the boundary, that is, their external and internal realities. In the English-speaking psychoanalytic group, patients make use of their exile (as a given), their mother tongues (so that they do not have to split off emotional responses and can really access their early selves) and the group as an 'intermediate area of experience' in a Winnicottian sense, and the experience of reality is made bearable.

Understanding in a group setting

How we experience ourselves and how we behave with others and with ourselves is dictated both by our conscious and our unconscious assumptions, which derive from earlier experience.

Christopher Bollas names those parts of ourselves that are unconscious and nevertheless affect us the 'unthought known' and contrasts this with the 'thought known', that is, our conscious memories (Bollas, 1987). All of us transform our earliest experiences with others into 'rules' which we use to orient ourselves in our internal and external worlds. For Bollas this is the 'grammar of the ego'. This '... structure of the ego is the self's shadow, a silent speech that is unheard by the subject until he enters the echo chamber of psychoanalysis. There the person discovers this densely structured grammar of the ego that speaks in the psychoanalysis through dreams, parapraxes, phantasies, and most especially through the nature of the transference ...' (Bollas, 1987, p. 72). In group therapy, one is confronted not only with one other person, but with several other people.

In contrast to the opportunity provided by individual therapy to enter into a relationship with the therapist in which the 'unconscious grammar of the ego' can come to light, in group therapy patients have to enter into various relationships with several other people. The assumption is that the many possible experiences of relationships and the protected, but also revealing setting of the group provides multifarious ways in which patients can expand their understanding of how they are with others. What free association is to psychoanalysis, the rule of openness is to the group. The group participants are asked to express as spontaneously as possible all that occurs to them, while respecting their own boundaries and those of the other participants. Special emphasis is laid on the group members' observations, phantasies and feelings about each other, themselves and the therapist. For the group to be able to work as a group, it must *be* a group. The main goal – both at the beginning and during the process – is therefore to create the conditions under which the group can feel that it is a group, that is, to develop good cohesion. This is the group leader's chief task – to protect the group, to give it a frame, rules and norms, which will then increasingly be sustained and enforced by the group itself. The group can only exercise its 'maternal' function of being a 'space to play' and container, a place where feelings, which are initially unconscious and usually strong, are 'digested' and given back in a tolerable form, if there is also a 'paternal' leader who attends to the adherence to the protective frame.

As mentioned above, patients who are in exile for internal reasons are often also traumatised. Their traumas are relationship traumas, which impair or eliminate their ability to find their bearings in the intimacy of interpersonal relationships. Most importantly, the group functions as a container. According to Fonagy, the maternal function of containing is the first mentalisation and symbolisation function that is internalised by the infant. Through containment but also through mirroring and resonance the group facilitates and develops mentalisation. The psychoanalytic group is an environment that is 'good enough' and 'maternal enough' to promote the development of the capacity to see oneself from the outside and others from the inside through empathy (Holmes and Slade, 2018, p. 66). That is what we call mentalisation.

It can help its members to tolerate the reality of dependency, limitation and loss because a space to play and think is provided that was not previously available. In the group, intense affects can be regulated and the capacity for regulation can be internalised. Group members can help each other to become aware of feelings that are hard to bear and to find words for them. Through mirroring in the form of identification ('I have experienced that, too') and confrontation ('This is how I experience you') they have a chance to make developmental steps that were not possible in their interactions in early childhood.

The patients in exile in my group therapy also show tendencies towards splitting – which is intensified by the experience of exile. Due to their loss of external safety-providing objects and the lack of an internal object that provides safety, they find themselves more often than not in isolation. Particularly those who have recently arrived might feel overwhelmed by the exposure to multiple new and strange impressions in the new country.

Clinical illustration, continued

About two years later – much to my surprise – Jill was back. She had found herself changed more than she thought and could not find her way back to her life in the US. Part of that experience, of course, was a repetition of the old. The 'old' country could not rescue her from her internal pain. She had not been able to grieve her many losses or to give herself the chance to achieve true integration in the new country. Yet obviously, something had changed. Not only was she able to return to the place she had left behind, she was also able to pick up the group analysis work where we had left off. In her 'second time around' in the group, she had a new role. She became the 'group's memory', able to store and relate every important exchange and situation. With this role, it was clear that she had gained a sense of continuity over time. In Winnicott's terminology, one could say that she was able to use the group as an 'intermediate area of experience' to gather and explore the various parts of herself which she had previously kept separate. She could then integrate these into an experience within a time-frame. The starting point seemed to have been the upheaval which her leaving had caused in the group. With their help, their minds experiencing and expressing something that had traumatised her, she was able to gain access to these traumatic, locked away experiences. This led to the development of a mentalising capacity, which has since then also helped many others in the group.

The deep desire for belonging is inherent in the human condition. Particularly in situations that underline differences, such as migration, we can perhaps persuade ourselves that we do not need the others, who are at once longed for, yet hated for their separateness. But, of course, we do need others. As in the myth of the tower of Babel, there is within us a longing to be understood, which is experienced as increasingly painful, as the reality of separateness is recognised. Yet reality is always a gain, a step forward from illusion. In the process, the phantasy of total understanding can gradually give way to the wish for closeness and intimacy within relationships in which the reality of separateness is recognised.

Notes

1. Translated by Deirdre Winter, Berlin.
2. A previous version of this paper was published in *Zeitschrift für Individualpsychologie 42* (2017), 196–204. Göttingen: Vandenhoek und Ruprecht, and is reprinted here in English with the kind permission of the publishers.
3. Translated by Deirdre Winter.

References

Abel, T. (2011). Zigeunermädchen – der fremde Bürger als Massenphänomen. *Zeitschrift für Individualpsychologie*, *36*(2), 162–73.

Amati-Mehler, J., Argentieri, S., and Canestri, J. (1993). *The Babel of the Unconscious: Mother Tongue and Foreign Languages in the Psychoanalytic Dimension*. Trans. J. Whitelaw-Cucco. Madison, CT: International Universities Press.

Bollas, C. (1987) *The Shadow of the Object*. New York: Columbia University Press.

Grinberg, L., and Grinberg, R. (1989). *Psychoanalytic Perspectives on Migration and Exile*. New Haven, CT: Yale University Press.

Hirsch, M. (ed.) (2008). *Die Gruppe als Container – Mentalisierung und Symbolisierung in der analytischen Gruppenpsychotherapie*. Göttingen: Vandenhoeck & Ruprecht.

Holmes, J. (2010). *Exploring in Security*. London: Routledge.

Holmes, J. and Slade, A. (2018). *Attachment in Therapeutic Practice*. London: Sage.

Steiner, J. (1993). *Psychic Retreats*. London: Routledge.

White, K. (2011). Praxis der englischsprachigen Psychotherapie in Deutschland. *Zeitschrift für Individualpsychologie*, *36*(2), 106–9.

Winnicott, D. ([1971]2002) *Playing and Reality*. London and New York :Brunner-Routledge.

Part III

Past generations, past worlds and the struggles of the patient in the present

The different languages learned in the course of migration can also be used as receptacles for different aspects of the self that remain split off from each other, so that the phenomenon of a lost, unmourned language can develop. This is also a phenomenon that can take place over the course of generations: a language, culture or country that was once the family home, but was lost and left behind after internal or external conflict. Thus it is that whole generations might experience the loss of a language and culture that can then be experienced as a hollow, empty space in the self in the generations that follow. 'Telescoping through the generations' in analysis can lead to a rediscovery of the lost part of the self.

Psychoanalysis has from its beginnings been deeply interwoven with experiences of migration and foreign languages. In a letter to Ernest Jones in 1920, Freud describes his struggles to understand the English-speaking patients, his 'entente people' (cited in Gay 1988, p. 388) whom he treated at a time when many Viennese people could no longer afford to pay for psychoanalysis. In the 1920s and 1930s numerous Jewish analysts fled Germany, Austria or other countries where they were threatened by persecution and imprisonment. They established new homes and new psychoanalytic traditions in the new countries, so that analysis itself became a story of migration in which its theories and practice changed with the move from one culture to another, with specific individual analysts leading the way in each country.

Chapter 6

The tale of those who went forth: on the inner experience of migration and forced migration[1,2]

Tülay Özbek

León and Rebeca Grinberg describe being an emigrant as an emotional state that is difficult to tolerate and thus subject to a wide range of defence operations. In the state of 'being' an emigrant, one exposes oneself to the psychophysical experience and must endure it. On the other hand, if one simply knows that one has migrated, one unconsciously uses one's intellect to avoid feeling what it means to be an emigrant. Rebeca and León Grinberg write:

> To be an emigrant, then, is very different from 'knowing' that one is emigrating. 'Being' implies assuming fully and deeply the absolute responsibilities that go with being an emigrant. To achieve this, one must inhabit mental and emotional states that are not easy to endure. Thus people need to resort to various defensive devices in order to limit themselves to knowing they are, without being, emigrants.
>
> (Grinberg and Grinberg, 1989, p. 66)

In what follows I shall attempt to describe these states that are emotionally so difficult to bear. Since the psychological demands placed on emigrants, their fears and their inner experiences of migration differ, depending on the generation to which they belong and the circumstances of their migration, I would like to try to convey a clearer understanding of this experience by giving a broad overview spanning three generations.

The first generation of migration

In the first generation the decision to emigrate is usually made independently as an adult, at an age at which the formation of the individual's psychological structure formation has essentially been completed. What I write about the first generation will draw mainly on the description of León and Rebeca Grinberg (Grinberg and Grinberg, 1989). These authors divide the process of migration into three phases and describe the different fears and coping processes that arise in each.

The *first phase* of migration is characterised by leave-taking, leaving and separation. Emigrants lose their social lives, their relationships with friends and relations, their familiar surroundings, and the smells, sounds, light, customs, norms and rules, and often also the languages to which they have been accustomed. These multiple losses initially result in regressive states. Renate Cogoy (2001) describes one of the specific manifestations of this regression in migration as the tearing of the symbiotic bond between the self and the environment. Quoting José Bleger (1967) she describes what he calls an agglutinated or ambiguous nucleus, an intrapsychic state experienced in early infancy. It consists of undifferentiated affects and a high level of uncertainty and ambiguity in which opposites and incompatible feelings occur side by side without this being experienced as conflictual or causing anxiety. As the capacity to differentiate grows and the personality structure develops, the ambiguous nucleus and the lack of differentiation and early dependency that prevail in it as unconscious memory traces are sustained and defended against by projection into the environment. This leads to the development of a symbiotic bond between the self and the environment which is the basis for the subjective feeling of safety and belonging and psychodynamically creates the subject's inner dependency on its environment. Cogoy describes how migration tears this symbiotic bond, since the environment is no longer available as a screen for projection, with the result that the inner world is traumatically altered. As this happens, emigrants experience a loss of the inner sense of stability that they had previously taken for granted. This can trigger primitive states of helplessness and they may undergo regression into ambiguity. Emigrants are often unable to get to grips with the real changes in the social environment brought about by their migration and experience themselves as being damaged internally (Özbek, 2015).

The shock of separation is followed by a further shock when the individual encounters the new, unfamiliar environment. These two shocks combined result in stress, anxiety and feelings of disorientation (Garza-Guerrero, 1974), since the automatic modes of adjustment to the environment acquired during socialisation fail because the ego is confronted with a foreign environment. The match between their adjustment mechanisms and the social environment is disturbed (Parin, 1988). On arrival in the new country, immigrants have to cope not only with loss, but also with powerlessness. The extent to which this loss is experienced as destructive is expressed in the term 'social death' coined by Mario Erdheim and Maya Nadig (Erdheim, 1982, p. 25). They describe the 'social death' caused by migration as a process in which 'the social and culture-specific roles disintegrate, the unconscious values and pillars of identity are called into question and with them the modes of perception that are adapted to them.'[3]

As a result of the multiple losses, being separated from their home environments, the 'social death' and the confrontation with a new environment, immigrants enter a state that they experience as a loss of self. Many immigrants of the first generation describe this as the loss of a part of the self: 'One part of me is here and the other part of me is there.' Something is missing that in the past they had always taken for granted. Chimamanda Ngozi Adichie describes these states vividly in her novel *Americanah* (Adichie, 2014). She writes of the 'sensation of fogginess', the 'autumn of half-blindedness', a 'milky web' and 'puzzlement' in which the immigrant in her novel was unable to see or understand the world around her clearly enough, a world that was 'wrapped in gauze' (Adichie, 2014, p. 160). The author also describes the shrinking feeling that overcame the immigrant when she realised that somebody was speaking very slowly to her, not because they had some strange speech disorder but because they had heard her foreign accent and presumed that she had trouble understanding (p. 163). And she describes the terror of the future that the immigrant felt when she did not know when she could return to her home country, her panic when she telephoned her relatives at home and there was no answer. Maybe somebody had died? Adichie writes: 'living abroad, not knowing when she could go home again, was to watch love become anxiety' (p. 187).

Immigrants experience these complex mental shocks and emotional upheavals at the start of their migration process, while at the same time having to dissociate them and keep them latent in order to remain capable of being active. Garza-Guerrero sees the co-existence of culture shock and latent mourning processes in the first phase as seriously threatening the identity of newly arrived immigrants. Were they to be felt, they would render 'migrating' impossible. In the first phase the wide range of defence operations that are employed in order to avoid feeling play an important in making 'migration' psychologically possible.

In the *second phase* immigrants must allow themselves (once more) to feel what they were unable to feel in the first phase. This is the only way to integrate the psychological shock, the anxiety and the grief into their previous experience of life and to allow it to become part of their identities again. Only then can they arrive and continue to grow. Thus, whereas in the first phase many of these feelings are usually still dissociated to allow the person to remain active, and the repression and splitting off of feelings is in the service of progression, in the second phase immigrants need to be able to feel again and integrate their feelings. Following a period of latency, the duration of which varies widely from one individual to another, ideally the memories of feelings that have been split off and denied resurface. Now the pain can be tolerated. As a result, the interaction between the inner and outer worlds becomes more flexible. In a sense, a new symbiotic bond is formed and the grief over the many losses can be felt. In this phase it is important to disengage from the lost objects and to be able to mourn these losses, so as to be in a position to turn one's attention to new encounters and experiences.

However, if suppressing feelings in order to be able to migrate turns into not feeling any more in order to avoid contact with reality, a traumatic core develops which is encapsulated in the self as a foreign body and must not be touched. To be in contact with reality means to be able to come into contact with one's own inner reality again and to feel once more what one has not allowed oneself to feel. This alone makes it possible, step by step, to regain a more realistic view of external reality.

In this second phase, which is also referred to as the transition phase, immigrants are concerned with developing a life space between what is their own ('I'/'me') and what is foreign to them ('not-I'/'not me'), between the group to which they belong ('inside' or the 'in-group') and the society to which they have emigrated or fled ('outside' or the 'out group'). Only when they are (once more) able to develop an interest in their present lives can they restore the continuity of and links between their own pasts and their own futures. If this transition, which is decisive if their ego development is to continue undisturbed, is successful, the pleasure in thinking and wishing and the ability to plan returns in the *third phase* (Grinberg and Grinberg, 1989). They cease to either idealise or devalue the past and what they have left behind, step into their current life space and then begin to inhabit it. Once this third phase has been reached we can assume that the grief about losing the former objects has been processed as far as possible.

However, if the person continues to split off the overwhelming anxiety and feeling of having been damaged and if the traumatic core is encapsulated, it will continue to exist in the self as a foreign body and the person will succumb to pathological regression (Grinberg and Grinberg, 1989). Grinberg and Grinberg rightly point out that the capacity to process the shock of migration is dependent upon the structure that sustains the shock – 'the less consolidated that structure, the more vulnerable it is to migration's after-effects' (Grinberg and Grinberg, 1989, p. 26). One of these after-effects is, for example, denial that one is an emigrant, which can manifest in the illusion that one will return and leads to psychological stagnation. The person is unable to engage in life in the new environment, accept it or take it in, developing a manic defence against the realisation that they have lost their home, those close to them and their language, clinging to a fantasy of returning home with an overflowing, rich and happy life as a recognised and valued member of society. In the first generation of Turkish immigrants in Germany this form of manic defence was clearly evident, for example, in their living conditions. The apartments in which they actually lived had to be cheap, were furnished only frugally with the bare necessities, while the real treasures were outside of their actual living space. They were either kept in the cellar in the original packing cases, ready for the big homecoming, or they had already been shipped back home, where one had a large, light-filled apartment, fully furnished with the best and finest furniture and electrical appliances – but those apartments remained uninhabited. On the one hand there was a frugal and penny-pinching life in Germany ('here'), and on the other a non-life of opulence in Turkey ('over there') – a fantasised life with a suitable life space displaced into the future in their home country – and a real life in Germany in impoverished real and psychological internal spaces (Özbek, 2015).

If migration is not voluntary and people are forced to flee, they are unable to make their farewells. They then lack the protection that this ritual offers. It includes both the hope of reunion and the possibility that this may never happen. In the period of separation and not seeing one another 'Goodbyes are the first thing one clings to with all one's heart and soul in an attempt to understand and accept the tragedy of separation' (Grinberg and Grinberg, 1989, p. 157) Having said one's farewells has a holding effect and provides protection in the sense that it permits the individual to tolerate the grief of separation. If the separation is sudden and the farewells cannot be said, this makes the mourning process, which is the precondition for coping with the second phase and being able to arrive in the host country, difficult or impossible. For refugees the transition to the second phase is often much more difficult because allowing themselves to become engaged in the new situation also brings up feelings of hopelessness, guilt and shame for having left their partners and families behind and betrayed them.

The second generation

The second generation are the children of those who emigrated. They have had to bow to the decisions of their parents. They were either left behind or forced to accompany their parents – and sometimes even sent back. At the time of migration they were usually still at an age at which the formation of the structure of the psyche is not yet complete and this fact alone makes them particularly vulnerable.

The emotional bond between the children who have been left behind and their parents is destroyed. They have grown up with surrogate parents, their grandparents, uncles and aunts. Being abandoned by their parents has affected the children in different ways, depending on their age at the time of the abandonment. We can assume that children experience the loss of their parents all the more profoundly and all the more traumatically the younger they are at the time of the loss. When their parents return home and visit them and they re-experience the loss this leaves them with emotional wounds that have lasting severe effects on their ego strength and relational capacities. A whole generation of children have spent a large part of their formative years without parents. Feelings of being unprotected, fear of attachment, and withdrawal are some of the associated emotional states. If the surrogate parents are successful in mitigating the pain of abandonment and helping the children to endure it, the effects of their broken-off relationships to their parents may be less stressful. The children who have been abandoned by their parents and then had to shuttle back and forth between their old and new homes are known as 'suitcase children'.

> M:[4]… most of them, I think they call us the second generation. They live in Turkey, are brought into the world, but most of them live in Turkey. There are many of them in my generation. There is *no attachment there.* And then at some point when you're eight or nine or ten, you get to know your parents, some of us even much later (…) then for some reason they send for their children to follow them. Then of course you get this conflict. *Yes,* because the children are actually wrenched out of their own worlds, whether that was their grandparents who have become their parents, or an aunt or an uncle who became their parents. … I didn't accept them [her parents], I said, 'Who are you? I don't want to stay here, I don't want to come here at all!' I saw my brothers and sisters for the first time. Saw my parents. I thought, 'That is your father, that is your mother'. I said, 'My parents are over there. … They've gone.' You are in shock.

This young woman lost her grandparents, the community and structure of life in her village, and her friends and thus the support and emotional security with which these people and this environment had provided her. Her own family was foreign to her. Thus for her, being reunited with her family meant losing her sense of belonging and security. There is no attachment between her and her parents. She feels uprooted and without ties. The many separations and broken relationships she has experienced since her earliest childhood have resulted in her feeling that perceiving and recognising her own boundaries and forming her own identity are difficult ('I think they call us the second generation – there are many of us – brought into the world').

> M: You don't have to be able to read and write in order to understand the life of another person or to understand his action(s). You simply have to be a person inside. People like my parents who have moved around abroad and have run around in miniskirts, some of whom participated in the hippie period, had cars or whatever, suddenly had *no* understanding for my generation or made *no* move in our direction. But, you know, an old man who comes from some mud hut in a village in the back of beyond – he says things that are simply human and logical and meaningful. You feel understood and can show even more respect for him because of that.

M's words reveal how deep the estrangement between these parents and their daughter had become, so that it was no longer possible for them to bridge the gap. She complains of having found herself with people who were foreign to her and had no understanding for her. We can assume that the parents' traumatic anxieties that were reactivated by the migration remained split off and encapsulated and that that made it impossible for them to respond to the deeply traumatic experience of their daughter in such a way that she was able to process her repeated traumatisation. Had they been able to, the external reunion might have become a resumption of their attachment relationship. It is my view that having parental objects who are unable to be empathic is the essential wound of the second generation. Both M's family and the culture were foreign to her – she experienced the reunion with her parents as losing herself, as being unprotected and at their mercy.

The third generation – affiliation to a group

I would like to assign to the third generation all those who have been born in the country of immigration. This can be both the children of the immigrants and their grandchildren. In Adichie's novel *Americanah*, the immigrant, Jane, tells us that 'this is my tenth year here and I feel as if I'm still settling in'. But then she worries about raising her children who might become something that she doesn't know if she is not careful. 'It's different back home', Jane says, 'because you can control them. Here, no' (Adichie, 2014, p. 137).

And Zadie Smith writes in her novel *White Teeth* (2001), of the immigrant's fears of 'dissolution' and 'disappearance' in the face of a 'legacy of unrecognisable great-grandchildren ... their Bengaliness thoroughly diluted, genotype hidden by phenotype' (Smith, 2001, p. 272).

Both authors describe the fears of a mother that she will lose her children and thus a part of her own body and her identity, to the new country. Concerns about a 'legacy of unrecognisable great-grandchildren' lead to the concern that one might disappear oneself, which in turn directly stirs up primitive anxieties about falling to pieces, disintegrating and disappearing.

If the nuclear family is strong and mature in the sense that it is able to contain ambivalence, it will be able to support its children in the phase of adolescent separation and individuation in such a way that children are able to benefit from the good relationships with their parents to become independent from them, open up to new relationships and develop their own identities. The culture of the country of immigration, which is in fact foreign for the parents, and their associated fears of losing both themselves and their children can be contained and tolerated. They do not then feel threatened by their children's participation in society. The children do not then have to avoid separating and turning towards the new culture and other relationships/objects in order to make manic reparations to their parents' impaired internal objects.

However, if the core of the family is unstable and beset by paranoid anxieties, every contact with the other culture is a renewed shock to the self. The parents' fears of losing their children to the country of immigration are intense. In such cases the parents' experience is not that they are releasing their children from the nuclear family group into the large group of the culture, or, so to speak into the extended clan, but that they are at risk of being lost to a 'foreign clan' (Erdheim, 1988).

For the children of the third generation, developing an identity and becoming themselves in the course of the adolescent emancipation process can then turn into a struggle with 'radical value conflicts and contradictions in the formation of ideals' (Wurmser, 2000, p. 25) and culminate in an unconscious conflict of loyalty in which they may experience becoming independent as a betrayal of their parents.

We can feel the panic in the words of one young woman whom I interviewed who described how she moved out of her parents' home before she got married. 'But I didn't violate the norm in any way! I mean, I still have things where I think in a typically Turkish way, too. That is, I definitely have, I can't think of anything, but I'm not typically German, either'. That she was no longer Turkish and had become typically German was what the Turks accused her of. Anyone who behaves in such a way as to break a group norm or calls it into question is simply not Turkish or no longer Turkish. Thus, for this young woman, the fact that she had left home before she got married was also tantamount to an attack on her identity. Since she had violated a 'Turkish norm' this attack was an attack on the Turkish part of her identity. She is afraid that she will not be allowed to keep this part of her identity and insists that she still possesses it. Since moving out fits the 'German norm' she denies that she is typically German. She is deeply ambivalent about the fact that she does in fact have a bi-cultural identity. We can say that the struggle she is engaged in is a double one: on the one hand the fight to find her identity in late adolescence and on the other the fight to assert herself and her identity.

But in the third generation this inner conflict and the conflict within the family expands to become a struggle with the majority society in the host country, since the majority society has difficulty in recognising the grandchildren of the first generation of immigrants as new members, that is, for example, as new Germans. While the parents of the first generation and those of also the second generation felt compelled not to let their children go, not to let them leave their original culture, the host country does not really want to accept them. They are repeatedly 'othered'. The 'glass ceiling' of racism is becoming more visible and more keenly felt. Millat, a character in Zadie Smith's novel *White Teeth*, says with bitterness that he 'knew he was a Paki no matter where he came from; that he smelled of curry; had no sexual identity; took other people's jobs; or had no job and bummed off the state; or gave all the jobs to his relatives; that he could be a dentist or a shop-owner or a curry-shifter, but not a footballer or a film-maker; that he should go back to his own country; or stay here and earn his bloody keep; that he worshipped elephants and wore turbans' (Smith, 2001, p. 194) and that he had no face in the country where he was living unless somebody who looked like him had been murdered. Only then would people who looked like Millat have their faces in the media. 'In short, he knew he had no face in this country, no voice in the country, until the week before last when suddenly people like Millat were on every channel and every radio and every newspaper and they were angry, and Millat recognized the anger, thought it recognized him, and grabbed it with both hands' (Smith, 2001, p. 194).

As regards group affiliation, the third generation are not able to distinguish clearly between what is their own and what is not, since they are identified with both groups (that is, with both the German group and that of their parents and grandparents), even though a feeling of being affiliated to a single group is described in the literature as being constitutive of the experience of identity (Erdheim, 1992). Thus, we often find that in their identity narratives individuals with a bi-cultural socialisation report that initially they took their identification as German for granted and that this certainty was only shaken when others reflected to them 'You are not German'. Belonging to both groups through identification is the basis of this generation's experience of identity, so that distancing oneself from, for example, one's affiliation to the German group is simultaneously always an attack on one's identity, that is, on one's sense of who one is.

While the third generation also feel German, the host society does not recognise them as such and repeatedly others them. This shock to their self-esteem brings with it many different emotions – the most prominent among them being anger and shame. According to Serge Tisseron (2000) the person's previous orientation in time and space is lost; shame has a disintegrating quality. For Tisseron, the powerlessness or impotence they feel is a mental manifestation of a breakdown that affects all areas of the personality, damaging the psychological, narcissistic and sexual aspects and cathexes and, I would add, since he understands shame as being essentially a social feeling, the social and symbiotic bond that the third generation had formed with their natural environments as a matter of course (Özbek, 2015).

What effects do this exclusion and othering have, coupled with the simultaneous demand that the immigrants and their children and grandchildren become integrated? I would like to briefly sketch some of these reactions and effects. The form they take depends on the psychic structure of the individual and on what mechanisms of self-protection they have or do not have. If a person is well qualified and is tired of being forced to remain stuck in a marginalised position in society, they may protect themselves from this type of aggression for example by re-migrating to the country of their grandparents. If people who are exposed to attacks, some of which can be experienced as annihilating, are not sufficiently able to transform this aggression they may act it out in violence. In this context the aggression of 'immigrant youths' (this label is still used to refer to young people who have been born in this country) against Germans can also be understood as a defence against their own feelings of powerlessness translated into what they perceive as power, the feeling of being a victim being projected on to the 'victim Germans' and then discharged in an attack on them.

Journalists of non-German origin, who have more resources that allow them to reflect upon and transform what they have experienced, 'shoot the s___ back into orbit' (Yücel, 2016) by making public the hate that is showered on them in readers' letters during readings of what they call 'Hate Poetry'. They feel that this is the only way they can hold and endure the hate and aggression. Whatever the case, something happens that Hasnain Kazim, a German journalist and the son of Indian and Pakistani parents, describes as follows.

> This debate has permanently altered my view of Germany, the country I come from, in which I grew up and which I actually also value highly. The people who came to the readings were presumably well-educated, probably have good incomes, and were at least well-dressed – and cheered their hero when he made extremely questionable statements about Muslim immigrant … I am of immigrant origin. The nature of the debate, this noisy pub talk strengthened the non-German part of me. I know a lot of people with foreign roots who have started to think like this this year. Do we really want to call a country our home in which people are met with such hostility?[5]
>
> (Kazim, 2010)

Kazim and many others reacted to the realisation that they did not belong by identifying more strongly with their non-German parts – they became more Turkish, Russian, Muslim or Indian after their unquestioned feeling of also being German had been shaken. Many of them reported that it had hardly been possible to talk to German friends, acquaintances and colleagues about it during this period. They described this impossibility of discussing it as 'not being able to get their pain across', 'not being heard'. But if the social bond is to be restored what is needed is, as Tisseron stresses, precisely the experience of being recognised by a witness, otherwise the rift becomes a rupture:

> First of all the social bond that he has lost must be restored. This bond unites the person who is ashamed with their opposite number, insofar as the two share the same milieu and are subject to the same constraints. In the situation of shame the other facilitates the resocialisation – just as he can, conversely, accelerate the disorganisation.
>
> (Tisseron, 2000, p. 13)

Identity formation

The result of successful identity formation is a stable feeling, and the subjective certainty that one is identical with oneself, regardless of time and space. Even when this certainty can be challenged, as is often observed when one grows older, or when one migrates, a person with a secure identity will always return to their underlying feeling of being the same, despite time and space.

I think that identity formation for the members of the third generation is extremely challenging due to the wide range of divergent identifications (Freud, 1921, Erikson, 1956) as these identifications take place within two symbolic systems and cultural codes with all the implications for the specific cultural characteristics of the psychic structure.

As described above, there are identifications with both ethno-religious backgrounds or large groups (Volkan 1999, 2005) and the matrix of identifications, leading to a feeling of 'sameness within oneself' (Erikson, 1956) is at least bi-cultural for the members of the second generation.

As Erikson (1956) has pointed out, identity formation starts where 'the usefulness of identifications ends' (that is, the identifications of childhood, in particular with parental figures) and 'as a subsystem of the ego it would test, select, and integrate' the identity elements, for example, identifications and self-representations. 'The final assembly of all the converging identity elements at the end of childhood (and the abandonment of the divergent ones) appears to be a formidable task' (Erikson, 1956, p. 71). I would like to add that this task is even more complicated if one is identified with two different ethno-religious backgrounds. As Erikson makes clear, 'the abandonment of the divergent identity elements' is necessary for the final assembly which leads to the feeling of sameness within the self. But growing up with and within two cultures can also mean that one is confronted with diverging identity elements (identifications as well as self-representations) throughout childhood. These can sometimes be divergent between the interplay between the cultures, but not necessarily within one culture. The divergence of identity elements emerges for example when a person has to identify who and what belongs to their in-group and who belongs to the out-group. According to Davids (2011), an awareness of the 'you', the 'other' as a member of the out-group, develops when a child is around three to seven years old. By the age of seven, the child is consciously identified as a member of an ethnic, religious and national group. Thus, an identification with the child's own group, the 'we' is formed, whilst unconsciously a negative identification is formed relating to the 'not us', the 'you', the foreign group (the out-group). When this development has been completed, the unbearable parts of the self can be projected into the out-group who becomes the 'internal racial other' (Davids, 2011, p. 57ff). Davids has described this as a process of internalisation that is inherent in the development of an individual psychic structure. This includes an internal object that Davids has named the 'internal racial other'. In my opinion, this process of developing an internal racial other also makes up an important part of ethnic identity.

We can assume that the internal object, the 'inner racial other' which is part of the individual's psychic structure, is shared by most members of the in-group. As it is shared by most of the members of the large group, it is the 'internal racial other' that ties them all together. This is perhaps what Freud was referring to when he wrote about the phenomenon of 'a number of individuals who have put one and the same object in the place of their own ego ideal and have consequently identified themselves with one another in the ego' (Freud, 1921, p. 116).

In the identification process discussed here however, it is not the ideal object that ties the members of the in-group together and with which they 'have consequently identified themselves with one another in their ego'. On the contrary, it is the internal racial other, the disliked or rejected object that ties them together. Freud, Volkan and Davids, with their concepts of 'identification', 'large group identity' and the 'internal racial other' were in fact, all describing the components of a psychic structure – an inner code – that allows one to identify the other person either as someone with whom one has a special connection as a member of the in-group or, on the contrary, someone who is seen to be the 'racial other'.

In his address to the B'nai B'rith, Freud outlined his identity as a Jew by naming 'many obscure emotional forces, which were the more powerful the less they could be expressed in words, as well as a clear consciousness of inner identity, the safe privacy of a common mental construction' (Freud, 1926, p. 274). He locates the 'psychical continuity' (Freud, 1913) in the early object relations where symbolisation is not yet developed and where only the 'obscure emotional forces' are the base upon which the 'common mental construction' is built.

One can say that the sense of oneself is built up on both: a sense of 'I am what I am' as well as 'I am what we, the members of my in-group, are – that which ties us together and lets us *feel* German, Turkish, Jewish, Muslim'. I think this is what Erikson determined when he defined identity as 'a mutual relation in that it connotes both a persistent sameness within oneself (self-sameness) and a persistent sharing of some kind of essential character with others' (Erikson, 1956, p. 57).

I assume that the members of the second generation have two ethno-religious backgrounds or to put it in the words of Davids (2011) they have two in-groups: the ethno-religious background of their ancestors' in-group (for example, to feel Turkish) and their second in-group, which is the large group of the land they are born in (for example, to be German).

However, both in-groups differ from the 'normal' characteristics of an in-group. Usually, as Davids describes it for the in-group and Volkan describes it for ethnic identity, it develops within the original in-group. But in migration, the original in-group is unavailable. The in-group within migration is a diasporic group. According to Mayer, the diasporic community is understood in contemporary social-scientific discourse as a 'genuinely new form of socio-cultural identification and interaction' (Mayer, 2005, p. 12). Stuart Hall describes these as 'new ethnicities' and emphasises 'a deep-reaching discontinuity' as a shared horizon of experience (quoted by

Mayer 2005, p. 11). Shermin Langhoff (2008) refuses to call the second/third generation 'migrants'. She calls them instead the 'post-migrants', because they did not migrate themselves, but they share a knowledge and an experience of migration as a personal and a collective/diasporic memory. It is important to realise and to acknowledge that second and third generation descendants are therefore first generation post-migrants and the 'foreign' natives, when they are born and raised in the land of immigration.

Normally one grows up in one larger group, that is, one grows up in the land of origin of the ancestors. The heritage and the personal knowledge of the post-migrant generation differs insofar as the land and the culture of the ancestors is no longer the country in which they, the descendants, the second generation, are born.

Mario Erdheim emphasised the possibility of building an ethnic identity that is decoupled from a region and instead is expressed through a symbolic universe. Such a decoupled ethnic identity can be found among first-generation immigrants who are far from their homes and home culture. It is this 'decoupled symbolic universe' that is conveyed to their (post-migrant) children in their earliest interactions. It is a detached, no longer regionally anchored, delocalised, conserved symbolic universe, which no longer experiences cultural upgrades. The process of regional detachment cuts it off from the social development of negotiated cultural meaning, which is usually fed back to the localised subject. What gets transmitted to subsequent generations is therefore a 'delocalised' large group identity, which gives the individual a certain belonging but also marks him as 'the other' who does not belong to the in-group, for example, as applied to Turkish youths who were born and grew up in Germany, meaning that they simultaneously belong to the large group of Turks, but their 'Turkish-ness' is nonetheless different from that of Turks living in Turkey. This raises the question of what happens to ethnicity and the 'common image of society' when, living in another country, there is no experience or feedback from the day-to-day reality of the former in-group. Whilst the former in-group continues to be anchored in the day-to-day reality, the diasporic in-group loses this anchor through the migration. The specific sense of belonging that is fed by the continuous, unconscious, collective feedback from the day-to-day reality to the psyche of the individual, is missing. Thus, we might ask whether the common image of the (former) society, to which the large group introject applies, does not become in some way illusory when, in the new country, the permanent collective feedback is no longer available.

The second ethno-religious background (German ethnicity by birth and therefore membership in the German large group), does not occur in the framework of early interactions with objects, so it is devoid of the pre-lingual and the sensual, and so the post-migrant youth, although born and raised in Germany, remains 'the other', because their 'German-ness' is different from the Germans who have German ancestors (prehistoric fathers). I assume that there is a lack of a primary identification, but due to birth and upbringing, a strong (secondary) identification. One does not feel bound, in the sense described by Volkan or Freud; there are no 'feelings and thoughts' that bind people without language to 'those that they feel, unconsciously and symbolically, to be their mothers or other important caregivers from their childhoods' (Volkan, 2005, p. 23). This feeling can only occur when one shares similar, early interactional experiences. Thus, the 'German-ness' of a young German with a Turkish background is always different from the 'German-ness' of a German-German. Nonetheless, German culture is familiar, because it is manifest in the natural external environment that serves as the framework for the secondary and tertiary socialisations that one grows into.

But Turkish identity as well as German identity remains precarious. One is neither a 'real Turk' nor a 'real German'. Both primary groups – the Turkish as well as the German in-group – can deprive the post-migrants of their ethnic identity. It was again Erikson (1956), who pointed out how important society's acknowledgement of the identity is for identity formation:

> It arises from the selective repudiation and mutual assimilation of childhood identifications, and their absorption in a new configuration, which, in turn, is dependent on the process by which a society (often through sub-societies) identifies the young individual, recognising him as somebody who had to become the way he is, and who, being the way he is, is taken for granted.
>
> (Erikson, 1956, p. 68)

So post-migrant children and youths have the experience that their (large) group identity is frequently not recognised as an identity of belonging by members of the primary groups, which is experienced as an attack on the continuity of the feeling of 'sameness within oneself' or perhaps as an attack on their group identity. The original group of the ancestors fear losing their descendants to the new, foreign group/culture. If often occurs that every approach and exchange between young people and their second, primary group is accompanied by a reproach: you become German or you are Germanised. Whereas the second primary group identifies them as Turks, Arabs, Koreans and not as 'foreign/new natives', they do, however, identify them as non-members. So identity formation of the second generation is very much involved and interwoven with a feeling of non-belonging (Özbek, 2017).

I am assuming that in the course of identity development in members of the third generation who undergo bi-cultural socialisation at least three group introjects are formed:

1 First, an ethnic, large group introject which, due to the history of migration is disconnected, is no longer regionally rooted and orients itself towards a symbolic universe that is mediated by interactional

experiences with parents, for example, for the Turkish immigrants this would be a Turkish large-group identity.

2 A large-group introject pertaining to the host country, which lacks early interactional experiences and has been acquired through secondary, extra-familial socialisation; for immigrants to Germany this would be a German large-group identity.
3 A diasporic group introject; I understand the diaspora group as an ethnically or religiously determined community that lives outside its original locality with its identity-forming narratives. Stuart Hall calls such communities 'new ethnicities' and sees them as sharing as a common experience of 'a profound discontinuity' (cited in Mayer, 2005, p. 11); in our example this would be a Turkish-German group identity.

I also assume that the respective large- and small-group introjects result in a 'diasporic group identity' which draws on the different group introjects while at the same time links them together. In my view, what links the different group introjects and at the same time creates a sense of identity is, in contrast to the situation with the first and second generations, access to one or the other or a third group introject, depending on context and changing over time, that is, an ability to switch effortlessly and without thinking between cultural codes. Thus, if identity formation is to be successful in several different cultural frames of reference it is essential to have the ability to bring them together while at the same time recognising the differences, which remain.

In my view, the diasporic group identity plays an important role in the process of linking and in the linking together of contributions from different cultures. The less illusory and split the diasporic small-group identity is, and the more ambivalence and ambiguity it can contain and tolerate within it, the more it will be able to link together the different group introjects in the subject in such a way that a feeling of being a self or being whole will develop.

Paradoxically, this hybrid identity is also essentially determined by a non-identity in terms of not belonging. In other words, only the recognition that one is, in fact, for example, neither German nor Turkish makes it possible to link the different parts together in such a way that one can recognise that being Turkish, Japanese or Nigerian is different from being German and that one's identity is hybrid, that is, German-Turkish, German-Japanese or German-Nigerian. One is not simply both Turkish and German, one is neither German nor Turkish, but a third thing, for example, German-Turkish. This is a very specific emotional challenge.

A hybrid identity formation that is successful in linking together complex cultural affiliations in such a way that the subject feels identical with itself across space, time and place is only possible if the pain and destabilisation associated with the fact that one does not have what was originally seen as identity formation, that is, a feeling of belonging to *one* large group, is bearable and accepted. Children of immigrants are faced with the task of recognising this specific form of not belonging, of mourning this relinquishing of a classical sense of 'mono-belonging' and transitioning to one of 'dual belonging'. I believe that in clinical practice it is important to acknowledge that this feeling that something is missing is a specific feeling associated with having a hybrid identity that is not necessarily pathological, or to consider carefully whether it is a manifestation of the development of a hybrid identity or in fact an identity disturbance. Being fixated on belonging and denying that one is splitting off the experience of not belonging can assume a pathological character. The aim should be both to integrate this real pain of not belonging, that is, of being neither German nor Turkish, while at the same time drawing attention to the fact that there is a new affiliation, which in times of transition is 'polyphonic' and 'dialogical' (see Özbek, 2012).

Notes

1. Translated by Deirdre Winter, Berlin. This chapter is a slightly modified version of a lecture given on 11 June 2016 on the occasion of the Long Night of Science in Berlin. The lecture was based mainly on an article published in the *Jahrbuch der Psychoanalyse Vol. 70* (2015).
2. A previous version of this paper was published in *Zeitschrift für Individualpsychologie 42* (2017), 216–28. Göttingen: Vandenhoek und Ruprecht and is published here in English with the kind permission of the publishers.
3. Note: all quotations for which no original English reference is given in the list of references have been translated by Deirdre Winter.
4. Interview excerpts were carried out with young Turkish women during research for my diploma thesis.
5. Translated by Deirdre Winter.

References

Adichie, C.N. (2014). *Americanah*. New York: Anchor Books.

Bleger, J. ([1967]1992). *Simbiosi e Ambiguità*. Loreto: Libreria Lauretana. Published in English as *Symbiosis and Ambiguity: A Psychoanalytic Study*. New York: Routledge, 2012.

Cogoy, R. (2001). Fremdheit und interkulturelle Kommunikation in der Psychotherapie. *Psyche – Zeitschrift für Psychoanalyse und ihre Anwendungen*, *55*(4), 339–57.

Davids, M.F. (2011). *Internal Racism: A Psychoanalytic Approach to Race and Difference*. London: Palgrave Macmillan.

Erdheim, M. (1982). *Die gesellschaftliche Produktion von Unbewusstheit. Eine Einführung in den ethnopsychoanalytischen Prozess*. Frankfurt am Main: Suhrkamp.

Erdheim, M. (1988). Adoleszenz zwischen Familie und Kultur. *Psychoanalyse und Unbewußtheit in der Kultur*. Aufsätze 1980–1987. Frankfurt am Main: Suhrkamp.

Erdheim, M. (1992). Das Eigene und das Fremde. Über ethnische Identität. *Psyche – Zeitschrift für Psychoanalyse und ihre Anwendungen*, *46*(8), 730–44.

Erikson, E.H. (1956). The problem of ego identity. *Journal of the American Psychoanalytic Association*, *4*(1), 56–121.
Freud, S. (1913). Totem and Taboo. *Standard Edition, Vol. XIII* (pp. vii–162). London: Hogarth Press.
Freud, S. (1921). Group Psychology and the Analysis of the Ego. *Standard Edition, Vol. XVIII* (pp. 65–144). London: Hogarth Press.
Freud, S. (1926). Address to the Society of B'nai B'rith. *Standard Edition, Vol. XX* (pp. 271–4). London: Hogarth Press.
Garza-Guerrero, A.C. (1974). Culture shock: its mourning and the vicissitudes of identity. *Journal of the American Psychoanalytic Association*, *22*(2), 408–29.
Grinberg, L., and Grinberg, R. (1989). *Psychoanalytic Perspectives on Migration and Exile*. New Haven, CT: Yale University Press.
Kazim, H. (2010). Integrationsdebatte: Sarrazins Sündenböcke. Available at www.spiegel.de/politik/deutschland/integrationsdebatte-sarrazins-suendenboecke-a-735774.html. Accessed 6 March 2014.
Langhoff, S. (2008). Die Herkunft spielt keine Rolle – 'Postmigrantisches' Theater im Ballhaus Naunynstrasse: Interview mit Shermin Langhoff. Available at www.bpb.de/gesellschaft/bildung/kulturelle-bildung/60135/interview-mit-shermin-langhoff?p=all. Accessed 20 September 2019.
Mayer, R. (2005). *Diaspora. Eine kritische Begriffsbestimmung*. Bielefeld: Transcript Verlag.
Özbek, T. (2012). Und es gibt sie doch die pakistanischen Cowboys – Überlegungen zur hybriden Identitätsentwicklung. In U. Reiser-Mumme, D. v. Tippelskich-Eissing, M. Teising, and C.E. Walker (eds), *Spaltung: Entwicklung und Stillstand – Volume on the Spring Conference of the Deutsche Psychoanalytische Vereinigung* (pp. 268–73). Frankfurt: Geber and Reusch.
Özbek, T. (2015). Phänomene von Gewalt in der Migration. *Jahrbuch der Psychoanalyse, 70*, pp. 141–60. Stuttgart-Bad-Cannstatt: Frommann-Holzboog Verlag.
Özbek, T. (2017). Living in Germany as a Kanak: some thoughts about nonbelonging. *Psychoanalytic Review*, *104*(6), 707–21.
Parin, P. (1988). The Ego and the Mechanisms of Adaptation. In L. Bryce Boyer and S.A. Grolnik (eds), *The Psychoanalytic Study of Society, Vol. 12* (pp. 97–130). Hillsdale, NJ: The Analytic Press. Available at http://paul-parin.info/wp-content/uploads/texte/english/1988c.pdf. Accessed 28 February 2017.
Smith, Z. (2001). *White Teeth*. New York: Vintage Books.
Tisseron, S. (2000). *Du bon usage de la honte*. Paris: Ramsay Archimbaud.
Volkan, V. ([1999]2000). *Das Versagen der Diplomatie: Zur Psychoanalyse nationaler, ethnischer und religiöser Konflikte* [The Failure of Diplomacy: The Psycho-analysis of National, Ethnic, and Religious Conflicts] 2nd edn. Gießen: Psychosozial.
Volkan, V. (2005). *Blindes Vertrauen: Großgruppen und ihre Führer in Zeiten der Krise und des Terrors* [Blind Trust: Large Groups and their Leaders in Times of Crisis and Terror]. Gießen: Psychosozial.
Wurmser, L. (2000). *The Power of the Inner Judge: Psychodynamic Treatment of the Severe Neuroses*. Northvale, NJ: Jason Aronson.
Yücel, D. (n.d.) Hate Poetry at Dortmund. Available at www.youtube.com/watch?v=R2_R9qDFC6E. Accessed 5 May 2016, starting at 02:16.

Chapter 7

Rites of passage in migration and adolescence: struggling in transformation

Cecilia Enriquez de Salamanca

One of the fundamental challenges in human life is coming to terms with the 'facts of life' (Money-Kyrle, 1968, 1971) of separation, differentiation and change. The cumulative effect of these facts of life during the 'internal migration' from childhood to adulthood in adolescence can sometimes lead to crisis. External migration in turn triggers the need to work through these facts of life on both an internal and an external level. In this chapter, the cumulative effect of internal and external migration is explored, with reference to psychoanalytic theory, literary examples and a case presentation. Where 'catastrophic change' is looming, psychotherapy as a 'rite of passage' can provide a holding and containing function.

Although in modern teenage life the typical 'rites of passage' that are seen in cultural and religious ceremonies or initiation rites have often been replaced by a more permissive culture that allows more room for individuality, the concept still might prove helpful in understanding the changes in external and internal reality when an individual is confronted with the experiences of migration in adolescence.

The expression 'rites of passage' was coined by the ethnographer Arnold van Gennep (1909). The term is used to describe initiation rites to mark the move from one social group to another and has developed as a field of research in cultural anthropology. The moves are marked by a variety of rituals that can be found in many different cultures all over the world and have been described as consisting of 'separation, liminality and incorporation'. These rites include religious ceremonies or initiation rituals such as the so-called 'walkabouts' in Australia, in which adolescents spend some months in the outback in order to make a 'transition' into adulthood through new experiences and developments, or the *Ulwaluko*, of the Xhosa in South Africa, in which the transition into a new life-cycle is combined with the actual leaving of the familiar home. Concerning the male initiation ceremony of the Xhosa, Richard Bullock (2015) has written that 'the *abakwetha* no longer actually go to the mountains, but somewhere close by yet cut off from the village. And the seclusion period is much shorter. When

63-year-old Bangile Pakamile went through initiation he was away for six months ...' (Bullock, 2015, pp 2–3). Prout writes:

> In the case of Indigenous Australia though, life-cycle stages seem to influence the motivations for movement ... the literature clearly identifies a peak in temporary mobility amongst young adults. This is the period of life when many Indigenous youth are exploring and contesting their identities in relation to the state, their cultural context, and wider social norms. Many use mobility as a vehicle for this exploration and to establish their own networks of relatedness and belonging.
>
> (Prout, 2008, p. 8)

In many religious traditions there is a ritual in the teenage years that marks their development from childhood into adult members of the church. In the German Lutheran church tradition, teenagers are showered with gifts and money when they are confirmed, to set them up for the journey through life that lies ahead. In South America, coming of age is celebrated with a big party ('La Quinceañera') when girls turn 15. It clearly marks the passage from childhood to womanhood, which in former times was an indication that the adolescent girl was now ready to marry. Nowadays, the 'Quinceañera' marks the point at which she has permission from her family and society to start dating. It is apparently a religious as well as a social event, mixing traditional rites of passage from the Indigenous Maya and Inca as well as the Roman Catholic culture of the colonial rulers.[1]

The connection between leaving home and the transformation of personality through a developmental journey can also be seen in literature, such as the German fairy-tale 'Hans in Luck' (by the Grimm brothers). In fact, many stories and myths combine the theme of personal development with a journey that is undertaken. In *The Hero with a Thousand Faces*, Joseph Campbell, the North American professor of literature and researcher of myths and legends, describes this combination of personal development with a journey in great detail. He calls such stories the 'monomyth' or 'hero's journey', and writes that they consist of a 'departure', an 'initiation' and a 'return' (Campbell, 1949).

These many traditions and stories show how the radical changes of the self during adolescence are dealt with by means of traditional rituals or in narratives. The changes in the self can be seen as part of the human condition. The internal 'migration' into new forms of psychic structure, object relations as well as self and object representations is an unavoidable experience. One can say that there is no such thing as a voluntary parting in adolescence: the adolescent is pushed into leaving his childhood self and identity behind both by forces from the internal world, via bodily changes, augmentation of the drives, and from the external world, that is, society.

Starting from birth, a child is repeatedly confronted with experiences of separation: birth, the weaning process, the move from infancy to childhood, from kindergarten to school, from latency to adolescence. All these developmental steps can be understood in terms of a 'migration' into a world with new external and internal boundaries. Arturo Varchevker (2013) wrote in his introduction to *Enduring Migration Through the Life Cycle*, 'an important reason why the concepts of internal and external migration are so important is that migration is linked to the concept of identity …' (Varchevker, 2013, p. xvi).

Particularly in adolescence, young people have to face the challenge of a 'migration': from the internal world of the inner parental figures to an internal world in which their peers gain a new importance. New internal landscapes and objects emerge in this process. The mourning of childhood in adolescence might involve a withdrawal of their libidinal ties from their primal objects in order to direct the libidinal ties towards new objects of identification, new kinds of relationships, including the development of a mature form of sexuality.

One could say that the migration of adolescents in this sense is never voluntary. Children and adolescents are pushed into leaving by decisions made by their parents, the wider family, society, economy and politics etc. Within this involuntary migration, they are totally dependent on the provision of a suitable new place to which they can migrate.

Insofar as migration is defined as a movement from one place to another, it also has a spatial dimension. The psychoanalytic concepts of the mind also include spatial terms, such as W. Bion's model of the 'container' (Bion, 1962), or D.W. Winnicott's 'potential space' (Winnicott, 1971). These concepts of child development imply that if the child's needs are met and their anxieties are contained by a primal object that is willing to take in projections of pain, fear and confusion, this will lead to the establishment of a protective internal figure, who can help the developing child to build up an internal world and a perception of the external world that is rooted in feelings of love, trust and gratitude. The concept of unconscious phantasy, which has an impact on every experience of relating to the outside world implies that external migration will always be accompanied by an internal migration. In Kleinian and post-Kleinian theory, there is a wealth of literature describing how the perception of a new reality will differ according to the kind of internal figures and scenes inhabiting the inner world, which have been built up through experiences of projection and introjection and the perception of the unknown. In 'A psychoanalytic study of migration', Grinberg and Grinberg (1984) write,

> The development of a human being can be seen metaphorically, as a succession of migrations by means of which the individual progressively moves away from his first objects […]. The oedipal conflict forces

> a new withdrawal from the first love objects, equivalent to exogamic 'migration' It then becomes necessary to abandon interest in the parental couple and go forth to find new worlds, such as school, new knowledge, objects and socializing patterns.
>
> (Grinberg and Grinberg, 1984, p. 14)

Development, on the other hand, implies a concept of time. Adolescence in particular is a time of vital importance in the development of every human being. It is a time of bodily transformation, of sexual maturation; a time according to Anna Freud (1937) in 'the ego and the id at puberty' of a 'recapitulation of the infantile sexual period' (A. Freud, 1937, p. 152). The second working through of the oedipal conflict in adolescence includes the introjection of a new physical self with sexual desires and the capacity to give birth. In the child's developmental movements of introjection and projection, constantly occurring between the self and the object, an internal triangular space as part of the psychic structure is mainly established by means of the working through of the oedipal conflict. The realisation of the parental couple, the fact that they have a creative relationship that excludes the child, can lead to feelings of loss, exclusion, depression, envy and hatred. Money-Kyrle (1971) refers to this as one of the 'facts of life', something every individual has to come to terms with in his development. The second working through of the oedipal conflict in puberty will also differ according to the various unconscious phantasies of the primal scene. In 'The Missing Link: Parental Sexuality in the Oedipus Complex' (1989), Britton wrote that the acknowledgement of the parental relationship allows 'triangular space' to develop:

> The acknowledgement by the child of the parents' relationship with each other unites his psychic world, limiting it to one world shared with his two parents in which different object relationships can exist. The closure of the oedipal triangle by the recognition of the link joining the parents provides a limiting boundary for the internal world. It creates what I call a 'triangular space' – i.e., a space bounded by the three persons of the oedipal situation and all their potential relationships.
>
> (Britton, 1989, p. 86)

If we consider that both migration and adolescence are each individually considered to be a time of crisis, challenging the ego-functions with multiple tasks and shaking the psychic structure to a maximum, then we can imagine what a radical impact on the psyche the combination of adolescence and migration must have. Such an impact might easily be regarded as a cumulative trauma, particularly if the migrating adolescent does not have at his or her disposal a coherent self and good object representations, developed through the introjection of a good, containing internal object.

If the migrating adolescent is haunted by a hostile, persecuting super-ego, the move from one country to another can only be experienced as a punishment, being driven out of 'paradise' (Grinberg and Grinberg, 1989, p. 5). This may well be accompanied by narcissistic rage and feelings of envy as well as a deep fear of punishment, that they might be driven into exile (again) if they make the slightest mistake. The result might be a persecutory object and a resorting to the use of primitive defence mechanisms such as splitting, projective identification, omnipotence, as well as an identification with the aggressor. In their book on psychoanalytic perspectives on migration, Grinberg and Grinberg (1989) discuss the potential traumatic impact of migration on the mental apparatus of migrants, leading to various forms of anxiety:

> The phenomenon of migration can trigger different types of anxieties in the subject who emigrates: separation anxiety, superego anxieties over loyalties and values, persecutory anxieties when confronted with the new and unknown, depressive anxieties which give rise to mourning for objects left behind and for the lost parts of the self, fusional anxieties because of failure to discriminate between the old and the new. Migration, in our view, constitutes a catastrophic change insofar as certain structures are exchanged for others and the changes entail periods of disorganization, pain, and frustration.
>
> (Grinberg and Grinberg, 1989, p. 70)

Much has been written recent in years about the possible traumatic effect of migration in the sense of cumulative trauma (Bründl and Kogan, 2005). Huff-Müller writes about the re-enactment of feelings of homelessness (see Chapter 3, this volume). Cohen (2005) describes migration as stirring up the question of where one belongs or feels 'at home' (Cohen 2005). The work of Salman Akhtar, who sees migration as a life-long transformational process in order to find one's identity on the basis of affect regulation, closeness and distance, temporal connections and social belonging is particularly interesting in this context (Akhtar 1999). One could say that the developmental task of adolescence similarly involves a transformational process to find one's identity on the basis of affect regulation, closeness and distance, temporal connections and social and cultural belonging. Since the pioneering work of Anna Freud (1937) who was one of the first to investigate adolescence from a psychoanalytic point of view, a multitude of psychoanalytic theories and literature on adolescence have been published.

The following case presentation of a twice weekly psychoanalytic psychotherapy with an adolescent girl from South America, who had quite a troubled infancy and childhood, illustrates how the patient struggled with her own transformational process, searching for her own female identity. Her two-fold developmental task of working through puberty and external migration led to a cumulative trauma. But in the course of the treatment it became clear that the patient's relationship to her adolescence and her migration could also be regarded as a two-fold 'second chance', an expression the psychoanalyst K.R. Eissler (1958) used to express the power and possibilities that puberty could provide in healing the wounds of infancy.

Adolescence as a transformational process, something you 'journey through' on the one hand, and the patient's four years of transitional stay in Germany on the other, came together in this patient as a difficult challenge. In this period of transition, the psychoanalytic psychotherapy accompanied the patient in her change into puberty. One could in fact see the psychotherapy itself as the patient's 'rite of passage'.

The patient had experienced a rather turbulent childhood with many 'migrations', moving to-and-fro between the various homes of her grandparents and her 'single' mother, who had separated from her father in pregnancy and who held onto the status of a 'single parent' even after she was married to a new partner. In adolescence, my patient had a further experience of migration when the mother moved with her to Germany along with her new husband. Using the concept of the 'rites of passage' one could see her stay in Germany as her 'phase of liminality' or transition that was accompanied by yet another liminal phase, namely adolescence. The patient was able to make use of her psychotherapy in Germany to promote changes in her internal world, leading to changes in her perception of the external world, as well as in her relationships and her identity. When her therapy was coming to a close, as she began to free herself from her persecutory internal objects and having achieved more stability within herself and in her object representations, the patient told me, 'if this is adolescence, I much more prefer it to childhood'.

Case illustration[2]

Two years after moving to Germany, just at the time when a large number of refugees arrived there, Alicia's mother asked for psychotherapy for her daughter, who was then 14 years old. She explained that her daughter was suffering from 'lack of self-esteem'. She tended to retreat into herself, said her mother, rejecting everything in the new country because she had not wanted to leave her home country and her grandparents. Alicia came in a state of depression and rage, conveying the impression that she could not bear the feeling that she had lost her childhood life, even though it turned out that her childhood life had in fact been quite difficult. She confided in me that she pulled out her hair when she felt stressed and had fainted twice after minor conflicts. Although her German was quite good, she was too ashamed to talk to me or others outside school in German because she could not tolerate making any small mistakes and then to be recognised as a foreigner. Even though her school was bilingual with many pupils with their own history of migration, A. and her mother had to make a great effort to become accustomed to the new European world with the differences in climate, food, housing, education etc. The stepfather was an employee of an international company and the family had accompanied him through the new work contract. As is typical for the child that does not migrate voluntarily, my patient seemed to have felt kidnapped by her own mother and driven into exile, just like the refugees, something that she experienced as a narcissistic injury. This was accompanied by intense feelings of shame and devaluation. Thus, she did not dare to show herself as foreign or 'different', as she was not yet accustomed to the new cultural codes. Later in therapy she called it her 'migration complex', feeling that she came from a less valuable country, that she was not perfect in the language and worst of all, that she had a mother who was incapable of providing for herself and her daughter.

The experiences of having to deal with a new kind of outside world certainly had an impact on the suffering of the patient. But after getting to know the early history of the mother-baby relationship, it became clear that the patient's complaints were also rooted in early object experiences which stemmed from an introjection of a fusional relationship in which the third was excluded. Making any mistake, or introducing a difference would arouse destructive persecution and exile in the internal world. On the one hand, the patient's self was forced to submit to this destructive internal object. On the other hand, she acted out her uncontained aggression. She perceived her move to Germany as an external proof of her internal 'expulsion'. Alicia expressed her destructive rage and her underlying depression when she commented that she was convinced that in her future life she would live in a dingy, horrible place, and would have a horrible job. Later in therapy, she talked about how much she suffered from the cramped quarters where the family lived here in Germany, how she felt she was tolerated, but not welcomed by the people here. In the sessions she absolutely refused to speak any German, rejected any offer to play with ideas, thoughts, repeating rigidly that 'it is not going to happen', and projected into me a deep concern that she might be suicidal and need to be rescued from her 'horrible' mother and neglectful German stepfather.

She continued to suffer for a long while. Often Alicia talked about how she felt rejected and therefore identified with an ugly, stupid being that nobody wanted or liked. Positive or hopeful interventions were of no avail, but only served to intensify her destructive comments. Because Alicia lacked the experience of a parental couple and had thus not been able to work through the oedipal conflict satisfactorily, she was unable to make use of a mental space, but seemed instead to be adhesively identified with her suffering. In the transference and counter-transference this adhesive identification was expressed by the patient's complaint about the cramped living quarters. In the counter-transference I was aware of a pressure to agree with Alicia, not taking on a different point of view. As mentioned before, it was interesting to note that Alicia desperately needed me to conduct her therapy in Spanish, that is, her mother- tongue, as if no further change, no more difference could be tolerated. In *Psychoanalytic Perspectives on Migration and Exile*, Grinberg and Grinberg (1989) write: 'Migration, in our view, constitutes a "catastrophic change" insofar as certain structures are exchanged for others and the changes entail periods of disorganization, pain, and frustration. These vicissitudes, if worked through and overcome, provide the possibility of true growth and development of personality' (Grinberg and Grinberg, 1989, p. 70).

Elaborating on Bion's idea of the 'catastrophic change', Meltzer (1988) has written,

> it is the new idea which impinges on the mind as a catastrophe for, in order to be assimilated, this sets in flux the entire cognitive structure [...]. If we follow Bion's thought closely we see that the new idea presents itself as an emotional experience of the beauty of the world [...] – Bion's formulation of mental pain and mental pleasure implies that the intrinsic conflict of both the positive and negative emotional links [...] is always present.
>
> (Meltzer, 1988, p. 20)

In Alicia's therapy it became increasingly clear that her mental pain needed containment. Although my Spanish was far from perfect, I began to understand that it was also this that slowly helped her: having someone who tried to understand and could tolerate her imperfection, who could not express everything with perfection, in short, a person who could symbolise the missing link.

Alicia called herself 'ugly', devaluing herself, rejecting the beauty of the new world, her chances here, the beauty of her body. On the contrary, she had to attack her body, denying her adolescent development by constantly stating that she looked like a 10-year-old girl. This might have been her way of trying to escape the fusional states and anxieties, holding onto a bodily difference from the mother, in order to escape the danger of repetition of fusional states in the transference. Meltzer (1988) has described the conflict and mental pain of never being in full possession of the object, always being in a state of insecurity. This mental pain was too traumatic for both the mother and the patient. For in the external world, Alicia had more than once been abandoned by her mother and then taken back as though she were an inert object in the possession of her mother. Alicia had been shocked when her mother decided to take her away (yet again) from her grandparents and to take Alicia with her to Germany. No doubt this was the point where Alicia felt like an object that was merely tolerated, a mere 'thing' for which her mother was now responsible, since the grandparents had become too old and sick to take care of her. In her rage, Alicia had threatened her mother that she would fail at school, not learn any German and be miserable all the time. As she had missed out on the positive narcissistic gratification of being a loveable, beautiful baby, her narcissism now turned into a negative, destructive narcissism leading to the symptoms described above. In the therapeutic relationship, Alicia tried on the one hand to form an alliance with her therapist. But on the other hand, she made sure that any positive thinking, any hope was attacked. Fantasising about her 'horrible' future life, or evoking distrust, distaste or disgust in the counter-transference were all means by which her destructive internal world was staged in the therapeutic situation. Thus, the patient held onto her suffering, her emotional scars and her missing links in a very rigid, forceful and radical way, acting out her feelings of being uprooted by pulling out her hair and making use of those parts of her new environment that were difficult or even destructive, thus not allowing the new place to become a 'facilitating environment' for positive development (Winnicott, 1971, p. 194). In the course of therapy, the patient talked about a 'toxic' friendship that she had formed in her first year in Germany. She also had refused to eat in order to make herself suffer and she said that she had dressed 'like a clown' in order to feel bad. At school she had allowed other pupils to insult her, feeling absolutely incapable of defending herself.

Facing her two-fold migration to a new country with a new language, unknown cultural codes and simultaneously to the unknown world of puberty, was probably overwhelming for Alicia, with too many radical changes in her external and internal world. As Alicia's childhood history was one of loss, confusion, missing links, leading to a fragile ego-functioning with hardly any triangular space, it was very hard for her to come to terms with the turmoil of adolescence, which Margot Waddell (2018) described so vividly as being '...'... temporarily stranded, as if perched on some kind of raft in the tempestuous waters of unfulfilled need, unfamiliar sexual desire, unwarranted aggression, and felt deprivation ......' (Waddell, 2018, p. 156).

With time, all the symptoms, the enactments, the staging of her inner world and unconscious phantasies could show themselves and be addressed within the treatment. Gradually, Alicia found her own way of working through the developmental task of separating from her primal objects and bearing the anxieties and mental pain of this task. Her identity diffusion began to change and make way for a more solid identity, starting with the realisation that she had a body which she experienced as uncomfortable, the realisation that she was becoming a woman.

However, when she turned 15, she refused to celebrate the typical South American tradition of the 'Quinceañera', probably because she was still struggling with the internalisation of her femininity and the acceptance of her female body. On the other hand, she was very sad that she could not attend her cousin's party, as she felt close to her. Her peers became more important, which of course led to a variety of typical adolescent conflicts, which were also an enactment of Alicia's difficulty in dealing with closeness and distance. Margaret Rustin has written on adolescence and migration:

> Adolescence involves a major and disturbing shift in identity – both in how one is perceived and in how one experiences oneself. [...]. He or she is thus not only taking up a new position in the family, but also placing him or herself in particular ways that shift and evolve through the adolescent years in the hugely important peer group and in relation to external social structures such as school, workplace, and cultural context ...
>
> (Rustin, 2013, p. 39)

In the course of therapy Alicia explored her family history, which was full of migration, poverty, depression and experiences of rejection. She told me about what she called the family 'identity' of being miserable and melancholic. Being left in the care of her grandmother probably implanted in the baby Alicia the belief that she was a substitute, a price that her mother had to pay in order to leave and gain freedom for her own development, for her 'migration' from the family. In a rigid society that was still haunted by the horrors of a past violent dictatorship, her mother too will have had extreme difficulty in dealing with her own adolescent rebellion and her search for her identity to find freedom of mind. Alicia had a 'second chance' (Eissler, 1958) to build up her mental space and to free herself from her fusional state by the same forces that had led to the threat of a cumulative traumatic breakdown, the forces inherent in adolescence and migration. In, *On Adolescence*, Margot Waddell refers to Irma Brenman-Pick's ideas that: 'The powerful forces and pervasive defences of adolescence may disturb or interfere with further growth; (but) they are also forces which make for the charm, vitality, enthusiasm and development of adolescents' (Brenman-Pick, 1988, p. 146 cited in: Waddell, 2018, p. 157).

For me this also seemed like a beautiful and helpful description of what was going on in the therapy with Alicia, over and above all the difficulties that I have described. Gradually, Alicia dared to show some of the more lively and humorous aspects of her personality in her sessions. She developed an interest in her own mind and started to study at school. Having found a certain distance, she could see and talk about the differences that she noticed between the lives and societies of her home country and Germany. She seemed to be able to use the geographical distance that she had gained through migration to build a positive identification with her home country, seeing the beauty rather than the devaluation. She could mourn her losses instead of enacting them. Then too, she was able to compare and to see the possibilities that the more permissive culture of Germany provided. Through her migration, Alicia was put into a new 'cultural context' which she was finally able to use for her search for an identity of her own. Her very difficult relationship with her stepfather also improved and she acknowledged his role in her development. Alicia enjoyed going out with her friends to the park, having the freedom and the possibility of moving around the city on her own, being aware of and valuing the open-mindedness in her environment to her ideas – in her teachers, the parents of her friends and her therapist. Sadly, the stepfather's work contract led to yet another move after the family's four-year stay in Germany. In contrast to her initial refusal to speak the language, Alicia was now keen to continue with German at a German school in the new country. She explained that her knowledge of German would give her some credit and make her more attractive. In my view this showed that she had found something to identify with in Germany, but it also reminded me of her typical adhesive functioning.

Although Alicia had found some internal stability in the course of her treatment, the next migration into late adolescence and adulthood will have confronted her with new conflicts. Her underlying depression and her experiences of rejection and loss could only be partially worked through in the therapy, even though the termination phase of therapy helped her to address some of the conflicts in a greater intensity. Saying goodbye in the therapeutic relationship gave her another chance to make a new emotional experience that stood in contrast to the ways that the family and the patient had previously handled separations. 'I made a scandalous fuss' Alicia told me, describing one event when mother decided to take her away from the grandparents. There was no space in her family to 'make a fuss'. Instead, the pain and the sadness and rage concerning the separation were avoided. In my opinion she will also need her adolescent vitality of the 'scandalous fuss' in the future, in order to fight against the impelling forces that are placed on her from inside and outside, concerning both of which she has no say in the matter.

Notes

1. www.britannica.com/topic/quinceanera.
2. For reasons of confidentiality, names and dates have been altered.

References

Akhtar, S. (1999). *Immigration and Identity: Turmoil, Treatment and Transformation*. Lanham, MD: Jason Aronson.

Augustyn, A. (2019). www.britannica.com/topic/quinceañera.

Bion, W.R. (1962). *Learning from Experience*. Maresfield Reprints. London: Karnac, 1984.

Britton, R. (1989). The Missing Link: Parental Sexuality. In Britton, R., Feldman, M., O'Shaughnessy, E., and Steiner, J. (eds), *The Oedipus Complex Today: Clinical Implications*. London: Karnac.

Bründl, P., and Kogan, I. (eds) (2005). *Kindheit jenseits von Trauma und Fremdheit*. Frankfurt am Main: Brandes & Apsel.

Bullock, R. (2015). A month with three initiates during the Xhosa circumcision ritual. Cape Town and Hoedspruit/Nottingham. *Africa Geographic*, *48* (May).

Campbell, J. (1949). *The Hero with a Thousand Faces*. Princeton: Princeton University Press. Third edition, California: New World Library, 2008.

Cohen, Y. (2005) Frühe Entwicklung und Migrationsprozesse. In Bründl, P., and Kogan, I. (eds) (2005). *Kindheit jenseits von Trauma und Fremdheit*. Frankfurt am Main: Brandes & Apsel.

Eissler, K.R. (1958). Notes on problems of technique in the psychoanalytic treatment of adolescents; with some remarks on perversions. *Psychoanalytic Study of the Child, 13*, 223–54.

Freud, A. (1937). *The Ego and the Mechanisms of Defence*. London: Hogarth Press.

Grinberg, L. and Grinberg, R (1989). *Psychoanalytic Perspectives on Migration and Exile*. New Haven and London: Yale University Press.

Grinberg, L. and Grinberg R. (1984). A psychoanalytic study of migration: its normal and pathological aspects. *Journal of the American Psychoanalytic Association 32*(1): 13–38.

Meltzer, D. (1988). *The Apprehension of Beauty*. London: The Roland Harris Educational Trust/Clunie Press.

Money-Kyrle, R. (1968). Cognitive development. *International Journal of Psychoanalysis 49*, 691–98.

Money-Kyrle, R. (1971). The aim of psychoanalysis. *International Journal of Psychoanalysis*, *52*, 103–6.

Prout, S. (2008). *On the move? Indigenous temporary mobility practices in Australia*. Working Paper No. 48/2008 Centre for Aboriginal Economic Policy Research, College of Arts and Social Sciences, The Australian National University.

Rustin, M. (2013). Finding out where and who one is: the special complexity of migration for adolescents. In A. Varchevker and E. McGinley (eds), *Enduring Migration through the Life Cycle*. London: Karnac.

Van Gennep, A. ([1909)1960). *Les Rites de Passage* [The Rites of Passage], trans. M.B. Vizedom and G.L. Caffee. Abingdon: Routledge Library Editions Anthropology and Ethnography.

Varchevker, A. and McGinley, E. (2013). *Enduring Migration through the Life Cycle*. London: Karnac.

Waddell, M. (2018). *On Adolescence: Inside Stories*. Tavistock Clinic Series. London: Karnac.

Winnicott, D. (1971[2005]) *Playing and Reality*. London: Routledge Classics.

Chapter 8

Psychoanalysis in exile: early migration in the shadow of the Holocaust and the psychoanalytic study group in Prague[1]

Ina Klingenberg

Psychoanalytic research on migration, particularly in its inner-psychic and unconscious dimensions is still relatively young. Grinberg and Grinberg's (1989) study *Psychoanalytic Perspectives on Migration* can be seen as the pioneering work in this field. The next internationally recognised studies on the subject were not published until roughly 20 years later, for example, Salman Akhtar's *Immigration and Identity* (1999) and *Immigration and Acculturation* (2010). Despite increasing globalisation and increasing numbers of migrants seeking psychoanalysis, hardly any further internationally influential monographs on migration and psychoanalysis have since been published. *Contemporary Psychoanalysis and the Legacy of the Third Reich* (2014) by Emily A. Kuriloff and *Immigration in Psychoanalysis* (2016) edited by Julia Beltsiou are two more recent important volumes in the field. Emily Kuriloff focuses specifically on first- and second-generation psychoanalyst émigrés and survivors of the Shoah, while Beltsiou's book is a collection of papers by various contemporary psychoanalysts and writers. Despite the importance of these works, the lack of contributions on the subject in psychoanalytic theory is nevertheless striking.

In fact, there has been a strong link between psychoanalysis and migration from its very beginnings. It was for the most part migrants who initially created and developed psychoanalytic thinking. Even if it is not reflected in their theories, almost all of the psychoanalysts of the first and second generations had experienced migration at some point in their lives, whether voluntarily or involuntarily. It is hard to find a psychoanalyst in these two generations whose history does not include at least one experience of relocating across state-, linguistic-, or cultural boundaries. Many analysts' histories include several such relocations. Freud himself had to emigrate three times: at the age of three from Freiberg, Moravia, to Leipzig, Germany, and a year later from Leipzig to Vienna. At the age of 83 he had to flee the Nazis from Vienna to London. Melanie Klein, Heinz Hartmann, Heinz Kohut, Wilfred Bion, Sándor Ferenczi, Anna Freud, Wilhelm Reich, Otto Fenichel, Alfred Adler, Otto Kernberg, to name just a few of the well-known analysts who are represented in almost every textbook for psychoanalysis, also migrated, in some cases several times. One can assume that migration had an important impact on the outer and inner experiences of these analysts.

However, there are few accessible testimonies of the emotional and mental upheavals with which the analysts were confronted as a result of having migrated. There is also very little literature on their own understanding of a possible influence of their migration experiences on their own analytic thinking and therapeutic practice. One exception are the quotes of, and interviews with, analysts published in the book *Contemporary Psychoanalysis and the Legacy of the Third Reich* by Emily A. Kuriloff (2014). Here Heinz Kohut's shift from the theories of intrapsychic conflict towards the theory of the development of the self is explained by the 'injury to his identity at the hands of the Nazis' (Kuriloff, 2014, p. xi). One can see that the forced emigration had a profound impact on Kohut, both on him personally and on his theory. But these testimonies are exceptions, possibly due to the focus of psychoanalysis on early development and 'inner' psychic aspects of the human mind such as drives, inner conflict, the inner object world and so on. Experiences of migration were seen as 'outer' experiences. Maybe there is a link between this and the suppression of traumatic experience by psychoanalyst survivors of the Shoah who disavowed the possible impact of adult trauma and focused on childhood trauma – as Kuriloff shows in her book. However, if we consider that the 'heart' of becoming a psychoanalyst – whether practising or working theoretically – is the development of the capacity to reflect on one's own inner world, including its unconscious dimensions (as Freud demonstrated in *Interpretation of Dreams* (Freud, 1900)), it is remarkable that the migration experiences of the early psychoanalysts left so few traces in the written world of psychoanalysis.

Today, in our everyday practice in the globalised world of the 21st century, we cannot avoid being confronted with the experience of migration. Working with migrants in the consulting room – as seen in this book – has shown us with increasing clarity that migration often does have an impact on the most inner aspects of a psyche. This does not mean that it has a traumatic impact – it can even have an impact that enhances development or one that is simultaneously disruptive and constructive. However, migration always has a profound psychological meaning, one that is both conscious and unconscious. In addition, we can assume that the impact of migration is in some way or another communicated to the next generations. This, of course, will also be true for psychoanalysts who experience migration. As analysts we are asked to be self-reflective, that is, to be aware of and sensitive to our own emotional responses to the material of our patients. This also applies to the aspects that concern migration. Since the history of the psychoanalytic movement is replete with migration experiences – our inner reactions to the material of our migrant patients might also be influenced by the history of our psychoanalytic community. It is highly possible that aspects of migration experiences have been passed down through the generations – from training analyst to trainee analyst – who then in turn become training analyst themselves. These aspects of migration may well have been communicated through unconscious fantasies and unconscious identification, atmospherically or even consciously. Work with migrant patients could touch on these fantasies, unconsciously bringing them back to life.

In this chapter I will not be able to provide an in-depth analysis of how personal life experiences can be passed on from one training analyst to another, although I consider it an important subject for further research and theory. However, taking an initial step in this direction, I would like to draw attention to a specific group of our psychoanalytic forebears whose members were themselves directly confronted with difficult experiences of migration, while at the same time becoming influential members of the psychoanalytic movement. They were organised in the *Psychoanalytische Arbeitsgemeinschaft in Prag* [the Psychoanalytic Study Group in Prague], whose most prominent member was Otto Fenichel. The group existed from the mid- to late 1930s. It was comprised of German Jewish psychoanalysts who had had to flee the anti-Semitism of Hitler's Germany and made their way to Prague, the capital of Czechoslovakia, which borders on Germany. In Prague, they lived for several years in a kind of interim-emigration, which meant that their personal and professional futures were highly uncertain. They were unable to return to their country of origin but could not settle in the new country, either. During the time they were exiled in Prague, Czechoslovakia was under the threat of invasion and occupation by Hitler's Germany. It would almost certainly have been a death sentence for the Jewish émigrés if they had not been able to flee the country yet again. Despite this constant threat, the group proved to be remarkably lively and productive, both in a practical sense as well as theoretically and politically. I will start by outlining the situation in which the group found themselves and then go on to describe their psychoanalytic achievements and theoretical ideas. I will conclude the chapter with a discussion of the possible links between their situation and the development of the theoretical ideas of the group within the historical context.

Flight from Berlin

After Hitler had been appointed Reichskanzler (Chancellor of the Reich) in 1933, the parliamentary democracy of the Weimar Republic deteriorated rapidly into a centralised dictatorship. Anti-Semitism increased dramatically and became more open and brutal. It quickly became clear to the Jewish psychoanalysts, and most of the psychoanalysts at that time were Jewish, that both their current occupation and their survival in Germany were under imminent threat. Only a few weeks after coming to power, Hitler began to issue statutes directed against political opponents and specifically against Jews. Laws, including the 'Law for the Restoration of the Professional Civil Service'[2] were passed that largely excluded Jews from working in the civil service and the liberal professions. As a result, three Jewish board members of the German Psychoanalytic Society at that time, Max Eitingon, Ernst Simmel and Otto Fenichel, were advised by their non-Jewish colleagues Felix Boehm and Carl Müller-Braunschweig to resign from their positions (Lockot, 2003, Mühlleitner, 2008). In November 1933, the Jewish executive board resigned and entrusted the board seats to Boehm and Müller-Braunschweig. Arguably, for several Berlin analysts this process and the unfolding anti-Semitic persecution was an important incentive to leave both the Psychoanalytic Society and Germany. Three analysts of the 'second generation', Frances Deri, Steff Borstein and Annie Reich, decided to emigrate to Prague. There they hoped to set up their own psychoanalytic study group (Lockot, 2003, Mühlleitner 2008).

Prague, a city of culture, but without psychoanalysis

Geographically Prague lies almost exactly half-way between Vienna and Berlin, which were the centres of psychoanalysis during the first three decades of the 20th century. Until 1939 Prague was home to a large Jewish and non-Jewish German-speaking minority. There were several German-language publishing houses and also German cultural and educational institutions in Prague at that time. In the period between the First and Second World Wars, the city was also considered a thriving metropolitan centre of the avant-garde arts, including the fine arts, sculpture, photography and design. Prague was particularly well-known for its modern theatre productions and its legendary film studios located on the Barrandov Hills, which at that time were the most modern studios on the continent. The art movements of Expressionism and Surrealism were drawn to Prague and were well received there. The city also boasted a lively café-house culture and a vibrant literary scene (Becher and Heumos, 1992; Mühlleitner, 2008; Šebeck, 2013). Prague's rich cultural life will certainly have been a fruitful ground for the young science of psychoanalysis. The Russian psychoanalyst Nicolai Ossipow was director of a clinic in Prague for a few years and gave lectures at Charles University (Mühlleitner 2008). A group of physicians led by the Czech psychiatrist Jaroslav Stuchlík, who worked in Kosice, a city in the eastern part of Czechoslovakia, showed an interest in psychoanalysis. Yet psychoanalysis had not really been established in the city before the Berlin migrants arrived and established their study group (Šebeck, 2013).[3]

The lack of interest in psychoanalysis that prevailed in Prague until the 1930s could be explained by the specific historical relationship of the Czechs to the Germans, or rather, German-speaking people. Until 1918, the Czechs and Slovaks had been subjects of the Habsburg Monarchy, with Vienna as its representative capital. Only after the First World War did

Czechoslovakia establish itself as an independent and democratic state. The majority of the people experienced this founding of the state as an act of emancipation from the dominant 'German culture' of the Habsburgs and of Vienna. The new state was intended to be independent of the cultural and intellectual influences of the German language. Psychoanalysis had possibly been too closely associated with Vienna to be received positively by the Czechs and the Slovaks (Šebek, 2013).

A psychoanalytic study group set up in exile

With this in mind, one can imagine that the society that the psychoanalytic émigrés Frances Deri, Steff Bornstein and Annie Reich encountered in Prague had not previously shown much interest in psychoanalysis. Nevertheless, the three seem to have quickly gained some influence in the city. They founded their psychoanalytic study group immediately after their arrival, as they had planned to do. It offered both treatment for patients and professional training for interested practitioners. It was also very important to them to pursue the further development of psychoanalytic theory.

Before going on to describe their work in Prague, I would like to elaborate on the personal backgrounds of each of these psychoanalysts. Frances Deri (1880–1971) grew up in Vienna, where she gained a PhD in philosophy and became interested in psychoanalysis. That motivated her to move to Berlin where she completed her psychoanalytic training at the Berlin Institute of Psychoanalysis. She worked as a midwife and directed a community service organisation. At the same time, she wrote extensively, publishing some 150 papers in journals. In Prague, she became the leader of the Study Group (Mühlleitner, 1992, 2008). Annie Reich (1902–1971) also grew up in Vienna, where she trained as a medical doctor. She first came into contact with psychoanalysis in Vienna through Otto Fenichel and Wilhelm Reich. In 1922, she married Wilhelm Reich and moved with him to Berlin (1931), where they had two daughters. In 1933, Annie and Wilhelm Reich separated. Annie Reich went to Prague with her two daughters and became active in the study group as a lecturer and training analyst. She was particularly active in the field of socialist sexual counselling (Mühlleitner, 1992, 2008). Steff Bornstein (1891–1939) originally came from Krakow. Her family moved to Berlin when she was about six years old. In Berlin she ran a children's home and presumably trained as a kindergarten teacher. Together with her younger sister Berta Bornstein (who later became a well-known child analyst in New York), she commenced psychoanalytic training in Berlin. She did this alongside her work as a teacher and became an important figure in a group of radical left-wing analysts who had gathered around Siegfried Bernfeld. In Prague, she assumed responsibility for the further training of kindergarten teachers and educators (Mühlleitner, 1992, 2008).

All three psychoanalysts were members of the German Psychoanalytic Society when they fled Germany. Within a few months of arriving in Prague the three women had already – in addition to their psychoanalytic practices – organised a training programme with a range of courses and regular meetings. Their ideas and the courses they were offering seemed to have attracted much interest among professionals in Prague and among other émigrés. The group grew bigger and made psychoanalysis better known in the city. A few Czech doctors, Emanuel Windholz, Jan Frank and Richard Karp, joined the group, as did immigrants from Germany such as Elizabeth (Lilo) Gero-Heymann, Edith Lodowsky-Gyömröi and Heinrich and Yela Löwenfeld (Müller, 2000).[4]

As early as 1934, Otto Fenichel – who was at that time exiled in Oslo where he established the so called *Rundbriefe* (letters that were circulated secretly among refugee psychoanalysts),[5] and who later joined the group – realised the potential of the group as a guiding and influential presence in the International Society of Psychoanalysis. In one of his first *Rundbriefe* he wrote:

> Under Mrs. Deri's leadership good work is evidently being done. Although the young group has not yet published anything, we certainly know their earlier works and views (Annie Reich, Steff Bornstein). For the development of the I.P.V. we consider that the admission of the group could be of decisive importance ... [It] would be very desirable that Mrs. Deri become a member in Vienna immediately so that she can propose the admission of the group into the I.P.V.[6] at the congress.[7]
>
> (Reichmay and Mühlleitner, 1998, p. 62)

In 1935 Fenichel himself joined the group in Prague and became its leader.

From the influence that this small group of psychoanalytic immigrants had and their productiveness, we have the impression that they brought psychoanalysis to the city of Prague with enormous enthusiasm and energy. At the same time, however, Prague itself was undergoing a change in its infrastructure and atmosphere. Between 1933 and 1938 Prague developed into one of the most important destinations for German refugees (Becher and Heumos, 1992). Apart from its geographical proximity to Germany and the remarkably liberal immigration policy of what was then the Czechoslovakian Republic, a further reason for this was the language spoken there. Prague had been a provincial city in the Habsburg Monarchy and was still home to a significant German-speaking minority that had been living there for generations. Franz Kafka – to mention the most well-known member of the German-speaking minority – had written and published in Prague in the German language. The city had a German-speaking infrastructure, with publishers, cultural opportunities, educational institutions and a German-speaking readership, and this had continued to exist after the end of the Habsburg Monarchy. Charles University also had a German-speaking department. These German-speaking institutions were naturally of great importance for German speakers of every profession in which language is central, such as journalism, acting and writing: 'The writers who emigrated through the Republic of Czechoslovakia included nearly all the well-known authors and artists of the Weimar Republic' (Mühlleitner, 2008, p. 268). John Heartfield, Ernst Bloch, Thomas Mann, Heinrich Mann, Erwin Kisch, Berthold Brecht, Oskar Maria Graf and many more turned temporarily to Prague as their place of exile. The city became a 'hub' of cultural and literary immigration (Becher, 1989, pp. 91–2).

For these German-speaking refugees, particularly for those more intellectual and culturally productive, the first points of contact were usually the café houses. There they could meet, exchange information, feel at home and discuss practical and intellectual matters. As in so many other European cities at that time, café houses were the customary and trusted venues for intellectual encounters. Hence, in the café houses of Prague the émigrés found a similar atmosphere to that which they had valued in Berlin, Vienna and other cities with which they were familiar. Here they could also find assistance with lodgings among many other things. Numerous refugees spent most of their time there. The journalist Wilhelm Sternfeld, for instance, himself a refugee, described the legendary *Café Conti* as a waiting room for emigration (Becher, 1989, Mühlleitner, 2000). Presumably, the psychoanalytic migrants were also frequent visitors to the café houses. They were possibly the first places from which psychoanalytic thinking spread into Prague, certainly they were important ones. Conversely, the arts scene in Prague may also have had an influence on the analysts:

> ... we had a very close relationship to Czech artists, because the Czechs, as artists, and writers, and poets were very close to the French – Apollinaire and other writers and poets – who were very much influenced by psychoanalysis ... As a result of this, many of the artists and famous writers in Prague were very closely connected with us and we had long discussions on psychoanalysis, art, poetry, and literature. The psychoanalytic understanding of artistic activity and creativity and its influence on them, was already thriving at that time.
>
> (Windholz, cited in Müller, 2000, p. 108)

Fenichel's arrival and assumption of leadership

Otto Fenichel and Annie Reich frequently corresponded, while he was in Oslo and she in Prague. Thus, Fenichel was well informed of the work of the Prague Study Group (Mühlleitner, 2008). He visited the group in 1935 when Frances Deri had the opportunity to emigrate to the US. When she left Prague for good, Fenichel was asked to lead the group. Fenichel had already been one of the most important and active psychoanalysts of the Weimar Republic in Berlin, before he relinquished his seat on the executive committee of the DPG[8] (Mühlleitner, 2008). When he was forced to leave Berlin, he first emigrated to Norway, to where he had been invited by a group of Norwegian psychoanalysts who had been in training with him in Berlin. He nevertheless followed the development of the Prague Group attentively, giving them his advice and support. He was aware of the potential influence that this 'progressive' group could have on psychoanalysis as a whole. (Mühlleitner, 2000, 2008).

Fenichel (1897–1946) grew up in Vienna, where he also studied medicine. He first became interested in psychoanalysis in his late teens and was accepted as a member of the Vienna Psychoanalytic Society when he was only 23. He moved to Berlin in 1922, where together with Wilhelm Reich he became a prominent figure in the 'Freudo-Marxist' movement.[9] In this context 'Freudo-Marxists' refers to a group of young and enthusiastic analysts of the 1920s and 1930s who set themselves the goal of integrating Freudian psychoanalysis and Marxism. Siegfried Bernfeld and Erich Fromm were two other well-known proponents of this idea. For 'Freudo-Marxists', Marxism and Freudian psychoanalysis were the most important schools of thought of the time and it was believed that by integrating them that they would 'naturally' enrich each other. In their eyes Freudian psychoanalysis was a 'natural science of the psyche' that was based on 'materialism' and made use of 'the methods of the natural sciences' (Mühlleitner, 2008, p. 186). Freudo-Marxists also considered 'materialism' and 'the natural sciences'[10] to be the basic elements of the ideas of Karl Marx. Implicit in their assumptions, of course, was the notion that 'materialism' and 'the natural sciences' were in themselves the most progressive means of developing insight and knowledge. Hence, so they thought, the combination of Marxist theory and Freudian psychoanalysis would generate the most progressive thinking of the time. Fenichel not only had a strong political commitment, he was also a prolific writer. He was certainly a charismatic and energetic personality. On his arrival in Prague the group became even more productive. He communicated the enthusiasm that he brought with him – at least in part – to the group. In a later interview, Gero-Heymann, who was also in Prague at that time, said,

> And Fenichel took it over, he took over the whole group and he was a wonderful teacher. Later on, I had seminars with Anna Freud, in London. Anna was a marvellous teacher as far as lectures were concerned; she could explain analysis in the clearest terms, but it was interesting to note that she was not as good at leading seminars as Fenichel was.
>
> (Gero-Heymann cited in Müller, 2000, p. 109)

He sought to broaden the group's range of activities and its influence – both within and beyond the psychoanalytic community. He fostered, for example, intensive exchanges with well-known psychoanalysts outside of Prague. 'Fenichel invited all the big shots from Vienna, who came to teach us during the weekends', said Gero-Heymann (cited in Müller, 2000, p. 110), while he himself travelled to Vienna at least once a month to hold seminars there. In order to promote scholarly exchange among politically left-wing émigré analysts internationally, Fenichel continued to organise the publication of the *Rundbriefe,* which he had started to write during his time in Oslo. In the late 1920s and early 1930s, when the political situation in Europe was becoming increasingly disturbing and radical movements were gaining influence in European societies, debates about political commitment also came to a head in the psychoanalytic communities. In 1932 Freud moved the two psychoanalytic journals *Internationale Zeitschrift für Psychoanalyse* and *Imago* from Berlin to Vienna because he felt that Fenichel and Reich were using the journals for their political, 'Bolshevist' (Communist) purposes (Mühlleitner, 2000, p. 219). Consequently, a number of Berlin psychoanalysts were worried that they would become more isolated from psychoanalytic debate and started to meet to discuss both political and psychoanalytic issues. In 1933 most of them went into exile and settled in various countries. The *Rundbriefe* were seen as an opportunity to continue their discussions and enable the members of the circle to remain in contact with each other. They consisted of letters circulated to all members of the circle, who were invited to share their thoughts, impressions and news, personally, politically and psychoanalytically. Fenichel wrote: 'The Berlin colleagues dispersed across the globe. We missed each other and at the same time we had the impression, justifiably, that an outside influence on the psychoanalytic movement, which was threatened by fascism, also within the movement itself, was more necessary than ever'[11] (cited in Reichmayr and Mühlleitner, 1998, p. 16).

In Prague, Fenichel immediately began working as a lecturer, not only as a teacher for the Study Group and their trainees, but also giving public lectures for a broader audience. His lectures were intended for anybody who was potentially interested in psychoanalysis, but in particular for doctors and left-wing political groups. Discussions with Marxists remained a top priority for Fenichel. He also organised lectures in Zionist circles (Müller, 2000, p. 113). Fenichel's paper entitled *Elements of a Psychoanalytic Theory of Anti-Semitism* (1946) would later be deemed by Jacoby to be 'perhaps [the] most significant essay ever written by Fenichel' (Jacoby, 1985, p. 143). This charismatic energy was passed on to the whole study group. 'Public lectures were something we all gave, at least the ones who were considered to be fully-trained analysts. That was for the general public', remembered Gero-Heymann later (cited by Müller, 2000. p. 123). Articles were also published in both psychoanalytic and non-psychoanalytic journals. As a part of the international psychoanalytic exchange, the group participated in the 1934 conference of the International Psychoanalytic Association and the four-country conference in Budapest in 1935. In addition, of course, each member had to earn their living by seeing patients in their own consulting rooms.

The members of the Study Group in Prague seem to have been in a state of permanent activity. Years later, Windholz, one of the Czech doctors who joined the group, remembered,

> On Saturday mornings we would start by having a Saturday morning seminar; we had a seminar on Saturday afternoons and Saturday evenings. On Sunday mornings, we had continuous teaching. Our whole life was made up of psychoanalysis. After these weekend seminars, we had three seminars each week. We would meet in a coffee shop and it would continue until midnight. Our whole life was full to the brim with psychoanalysis ...
>
> (Windholz, cited in Müller, 2000, p. 113)

They seem to have applied themselves tirelessly to their own psychoanalytic thinking and to discussions of their psychoanalytic theory-building. It is likely that the enthusiasm and way of life of these exiled psychoanalysts had a positive influence on the reception of psychoanalysis in the Prague society. In any event, novels set in Prague of the 1930s and 1940s contain numerous references to psychoanalysis which was clearly well-known at this point and had become integrated into Czech society as a whole (Anastas, 2005, Weil, 1992).

The Prague Group's 'materialist-psychoanalytic' opposition to the theory of the death drive: an attempt to deny the real death threat?

Fenichel had, as mentioned above, emphatically sought an exchange with the political representatives of Marxism. This interdisciplinary exchange was important for him because he saw psychoanalysis as 'complementary to the emancipatory goals of the Marxist theory of society' (Schneider, 1999). He considered himself a Marxist. As mentioned above, 'Freudo-Marxism' had already emerged in the 1920s in Berlin. Many Berlin psychoanalysts – Karen Horney, for example, sympathised with these ideas, at least for a while. To be revolutionary, free-spirited and open to new and off-beat ideas was part of the Berlin *Zeitgeist* of the Weimar Republic and psychoanalysis and Marxism were indeed unorthodox and revolutionary at that time. It seems, however, that in Prague, the émigrés' commitment to Marxism became even stronger and their arguments eventually also became more oriented towards discussing Freud's new theory of the death drive.

In Prague, Fenichel sought to attract 'good Marxists for the complete education of the psychoanalyst' and to further pursue his project of bringing Marxism and psychoanalysis together toward a theory of the present (see Schneider, 1999). Prior to his arrival in Prague, he had already, step-by-step, been instrumental in establishing a 'working group of analysts and Marxists'. In the *Rundbriefe* we read that '... the working group of analysts and Marxists in Prague has now [*c*.1935] come into being and organized three evenings' (Müller, 2000, p. 131). The members of the group were psychoanalysts and Marxists who met regularly in order to discuss texts on social theory by Friedrich Engels and Max Weber, among others. Some members of the group published articles in socialist journals or held public lectures on the subject of Marxism and psychoanalysis. 'In both cases [i.e. at two meetings] there was a very stimulating discussion ...' (Reichmayr and Mühlleitner, 1998, pp. 182–3). Prague seemed to offer a fruitful ground for the exchange between analysts and Marxists.

After 1933 the city also became a preferred destination for refugees who were active Social Democrats and Communists, and their organisations. For example, as early as June 1933 the SDP (Socialist Democratic Party Germany) had established party headquarters in Prague and other institutions of left-wing activist groups such as Communists and trade unionists followed. Left-wing journals were published in Prague and smuggled into the German 'Reich' (Becher, 1989, pp. 39–40). Points of contact between analysts and left-wing political activists were thus manifold. The fact that both groups were in exile will have engendered a feeling of solidarity and closeness. Perhaps the immigrant analysts, or at least some of them, felt a moral pressure to turn to Marxism and to incorporate it into their analytical thinking. At the time in some left-wing circles it was important to be a Marxist or a socialist and this was considered to be substantial evidence of progressive thinking, perhaps as a badge denoting one's refusal to collaborate with fascists or the Nazis. In the 1970s, Henry Löwenfeld wrote to Margarete and Alexander Mitscherlich: 'I can see how difficult it was back then in Prague among the emigrants not to be a faithful Marxist, Communist, S.A.P., social democrat or Trotskyist' (Mitscherlich-Archiv Frankfurt am Main, cited in Müller, 2000, p. 130). Certainly, for Fenichel and his inner circle, their relationship to Marxism had become a central issue, around which the value of psychoanalysis revolved. The resoluteness of the arguments and the terminology used in several articles in Fenichel's *Rundbriefe* bear vivid testament to this, for example, '... that we press ahead with psychoanalysis as a natural science, i.e. with Marxist, dialectical-materialist psychoanalysis and are determined ...', and Fenichel continued pugnaciously 'to defend it, even against Freud, insofar as he has become inconsistent' (Reichmayr and Mühlleitner, 1998, p. 90).

The Marxist elements that were held to be indispensable for psychoanalysis were its critique of bourgeois society and the materialist, or dialectic-materialistic conceptualisation of science. Psychological suffering and the development of neuroses were considered to result just as much from problems in bourgeois society as from the inner dynamics of the human mind – this was the understanding that prevailed in the group. The two were thought to influence each other in a 'dialectical' process. The view was that psychoanalytic dilettantism in regard to social analysis (Schneider, 1999) would therefore need to be overcome to allow analysis to develop further, both theoretically and clinically. Conversely, society must undergo revolutionary change to better enable the individual to free themselves from their neuroses, or rather, for these not to emerge in the first place. Yet still more important than the Marxist critique of society was Fenichel's and his followers' understanding of the Marxist definition of science. Theory, in their eyes, was only 'progressive' and contemporary if it was 'materialist'. 'Materialist' was in turn used synonymously with the term, 'science'. In the view of the Prague Group psychoanalysis was 'materialistic' since it was based primarily on the Freudian theory of instincts. This was 'materialistic' because it was based on empirical observation by Freud in his practice, and because it showed that the psyche, the mind, is derived from the soma, the body. In Freud's psychoanalysis the instincts are seen as the link between the body and the psyche. This postulated link was seen by the Freudian Marxists as the equivalent to Karl Marx's famous credo 'Das Sein bestimmt das Bewusstsein', or, 'it is not the consciousness of men that determines their being, but on the contrary their social being that determines their consciousness' (Marx [1859]2010, p. 160). This is frequently seen as the core sentence of materialistic thinking. For the Freudo-Marxists instinct theory consequently became the core of 'materialist' psychoanalysis. What was meant by 'instinct theory', however, was only Freud's early theory of the libido. Freud's theory of the death instinct as developed in 1920 was rigorously opposed by the Prague Group, who described it as a 'metaphysical mistaken fantasy' (Reichmayer and Mühlleitner, 1998, p. 95) Moreover, anything 'metaphysical' was seen as being negative and 'reactionary' because according to the Marxists it was hostile to progress and potentially affirmed the prevailing 'bourgeois' and 'fascist' society. The Group argued against the death instinct as energetically as they defended the theory of dialectical materialism. In one of the first *Rundbriefe*, György Gerö wrote,

> Since the [introduction of] the doctrine of the death instinct an increasingly pronounced deviation from the revolutionary empirical findings of psychoanalysis has been perceptible. The original formula that neuroses arise from the clash of childhood instincts with the inhibiting powers of society has been abandoned and replaced by theories about a need for punishment, the weakness of the infantile ego, etc., etc.. Scientifically oriented psychoanalysis is based on empirical observations and this is clearest in the libido theory. The opposition group [the group organised

> by Fenichel] wanted to protect this scientifically oriented psychoanalysis from metaphysical deviations in order to be able to continue to focus on expanding on it.[12]
>
> (Gerö, cited in Reichmayr and Mühlleitner, 1998, p. 86)

And somewhat later, referring to the function of taking the critical stance towards society that was expected of psychoanalysis,

> Moreover, the opposition group finds that psychoanalysis is no longer fulfilling its function of criticising and grappling with culture. Those clear and bold sentences which we find, for instance, in Freud's essay entitled 'Civilized Sexual Morality and Modern Nervous Illness' and which implicitly contain within them an entire programme of the cultural criticism that originated in psychoanalysis have been forgotten.[13]
>
> (Reichmayer and Mühlleitner 1998, pp. 86–7)

The political and psychoanalytical positions within the Prague group were not, of course, homogenous. Gerö criticised Fenichel in a letter published in the *Rundbriefe*.

> You limit yourself too much to criticism and offer too little that is positive in its place. To me it seems that the most important task consists primarily in making those in the IPA who are not completely stupefied ... aware that they have imbecilically confused world affairs with therapy sessions, which is the mistake that most psychoanalysts make. At the same time, we do not have to interpret reality directly in the way that Marxism does.[14]
>
> (Gerö, cited by Müller, 2000, p. 115)

And Gero-Heymann stated that, 'Fenichel was more or less a Marxist. I had nothing to do with that. I was anti-Nazi and for democracy, but not communist ...' (cited in Mueller, 2000, p. 114). However, there can be no doubt that the attitude of its members towards the Marxist critique of society played an important role in the identity of the Prague group.

In the Europe of the 1920s and 1930s Marxism, Communism and socialism were to be found not only among the left-wing working-classes, but also in intellectual and cultural circles in which socially enlightened and progressive ideas were discussed. Is seems to have been a matter of substantial importance to the group that they were 'progressive', forward-looking and morally on the side of the 'oppressed' rather the on the side of the 'oppressors'.

In the particularly difficult situation of exile, that is, of forced migration, where they were faced with a highly uncertain future, the constant threat of German occupation, the impossibility of returning to their home country and concerns for friends and relatives whom they had left behind in Germany, the fierce and apparently inflexible defence of Marxism may well have served the members of the group as a kind of self-reassurance, a strengthening of their own identity, even a reassurance of their own right to exist. Although they may not have discussed it often, it was a fact that their right to exist had been openly called into question by the National Socialists in Germany and elsewhere. Nearly all of the psychoanalysts in Prague at the time were Jewish. In Germany, an expansive fascist movement, one for which expulsion and the annihilation of all Jews was a fixed policy, had gained real 'materialised' power. Even if the Jewish psychoanalysts in Prague in the 1930s were not themselves imminently threatened with death, this was certainly the case for relatives who had remained in Germany. The constant threat of German invasion served to heighten their fears of annihilation and those who did manage to escape later experienced survivor guilt.

On the other hand, with the founding of the Soviet Union in 1917, Communism had also shown real 'materialised' state power. In diverse European countries there were Communist, socialist and social democratic parties and groups with money and weapons at their disposal who understood themselves as anti-fascist. 'Marxism' and everything associated with it was perhaps considered, perhaps unconsciously, to be the sole effective opposition to National Socialism and Fascism, so that numerous hopes and conscious and unconscious phantasies were attached to these philosophies and political movements. In the psychodynamic structure proximity to, or identification, even an unconscious imagined merging, with powers opposed to National Socialism may have served as a defence mechanism against the existential fear and the real threat of elimination. If writings were labelled 'Marxist' or 'materialist', they were accorded a higher value. Thus Freud's early libido theory was vehemently defended, also because it was seen as 'materialist' and therefore implicitly Marxist. In the first letter of the *Rundbriefe,* Fenichel wrote,

> We are all convinced that we can recognize in Freud's psychoanalysis the germ of a future dialectical materialist psychology, and that there is therefore an urgent need to nurture and develop this science. If we did not believe that, we would not be psychoanalysts by profession. We continue to believe that nurture and development – in response to the resistance with which psychoanalysis meets for well-known reasons – is best done through working groups that seek to do positive work undisturbed by external resistance.
>
> (Reichmayr and Mühlleitner, 1998, p. 35)[15]

This passage can be seen as defining one of the key missions of Fenichel and his Study Group in Prague.

The death-instinct theory soon became a major subject of debate, paralleling the significance of Marxism for psychoanalysis. At the 1935 *Vierländertagung* [Four countries conference] for psychoanalysis which included Austria, Italy, Hungary and Czechoslovakia), the discussion of the death drive was the main topic, alongside the pressing current political questions. For this conference, Fenichel wrote a paper entitled *Zur Kritik des Todestriebes* [A Critique of the Death Instinct]. In the *Rundbriefe* he contributed an exhaustive discussion of the topic in which he compared Freud's, Reich's and his own understanding of the death drive, stating that, 'Instinct is the concept that is used to describe our biological needs, and it is thus the indispensable bridge between our science and biology. ... The death instinct does not fit such a definition of the instinct'[16] (Reichmayr and Mühlleitner, 1998, p. 816). This questioned the scientific 'materialist' basis of the theory of the death instinct, thus implying that it was non-Marxist. As I have already shown, Fenichel saw the main task of the Prague Study Group as helping to 'protect' psychoanalysis from those 'mistaken metaphysical fantasies'. At the end of his discussion in the *Rundbriefe* he concluded: 'I am against making the issue of whether you believe in the death instinct the sole and decisive shibboleth, the banner of psychoanalysis'[17] (Reichmayr and Mühlleitner, 1998, p. 820). Fenichel's discussion in the *Rundbriefe* suggests that he assiduously considered different aspects of the theory of the death instinct, but his choice of words also appears to show that the question of the death instinct was close to becoming, or already was, a shibboleth, or, in other words, a creed. 'Either you believe in the death instinct, or you don't belong to the psychoanalytic movement'. Otherwise Fenichel would not have needed to point it up in this way. At all events, the theory of the death drive seemed to combine all that was considered to be 'bad' by the Prague Group. They deemed it 'metaphysical', 'not materialistic', 'not Marxist' and 'not naturally scientific' and therefore an endorsement of social oppression. There was a tacit understanding that it cast doubt on the theory of the sex instinct and on belief in positive life forces.

Certainly, over the years Freud's theory of the death instinct, and its further development by Melanie Klein, has frequently sparked heated discussions and provoked fierce rejections, even total disregard, and continues to do so today. In her *Preface* to the German edition[18] of the writings of Melanie Klein,[19] Ruth Cycon (1995) describes how in Germany, for example, Melanie Klein's insights and thoughts were ignored for decades after the Second World War and the Shoah, '[it is] inconceivable that ... the theories of Melanie Klein could have been discussed at that time – at least in Germany – in a way that could have led to a differentiated exploration of destructive narcissism, psychotic fears and omnipotent defence mechanisms'[20] (Cycon, 1995, p. xiii). For the émigré analysts who lived in Prague from 1933–1938, the rejection of the death instinct and the energy they invested in the debate about it, probably took on the function of an unconscious psychodynamic defence. In its substance the theory of the death instinct threatened to shatter the unconscious hopes that they had placed in a positive life-sustaining power, a hope that Marxism seems to have represented for them, helping them to mentally survive this period of utter uncertainty and loss. Marxism and Freud's early drive theory may have provided a theoretically 'proven' foundation for this hope and helped them to sustain the unconscious fantasy of a rescuing power that might eventually prevail.

After the German invasion of Czechoslovakia in 1938, all Jewish psychoanalysts were imminently threatened with incarceration in concentration camps and death. By then Fenichel and a couple of other analysts had already received an 'Ausreiseaufforderung', (an order to leave the country), from the Czechoslovakian state and had taken measures to leave. Now leaving had become a matter of survival. Whoever could, tried to emigrate. Most eventually went to the US. As far as I know, after this second emigration to the US, none of the analysts who had attributed such a central role to Marxism continued to do so – at least in public. There were certainly many reasons for this, one being the American anti-Communist stance at that time, but also the conditions which the immigrants had to fulfil and their struggle to settle down in the new country. One further reason could well have been the sense that Marxism as a protective and progressive force, which had served them as an intra-psychic defence in the face of the threat of Nazi terror and death, could now be given up. Finally, in their new home country that threat no longer existed.

Some concluding observations

Despite the manifold experiences of migration that many members of the psychoanalytic community have had since the beginning of psychoanalysis, the impact of migration on the psyche has only recently become a topic of psychoanalytic research. These studies show that migration always involves a number of challenges which, depending on the individual's mental capacities and the specific circumstances of the migration, may or may not be mastered satisfactorily. While these challenges can result in mental breakdown, they can also lead to development and growth. Migration always involves a loss and separation from what is familiar, and always requires an internal upheaval to accommodate what is new. Grinberg and Grinberg have shown that many different fears are triggered, with corresponding defence reactions and symptoms, which can then lead to a 'psychopathology of migration' (Grinberg and Grinberg, 1989, p. 1), in which the integrity of the ego is felt to be at least temporarily threatened. Akhtar identifies multiple factors that contribute to the emotional stress of the migration experience. Is the migration voluntary or involuntary, temporary or lasting, sudden or planned, thus allowing for an anticipatory mourning? Can the country of origin be visited (to 'refuel' emotionally)? Was the person forced to migrate to escape persecution, or were they searching for new horizons?

Bearing these factors in mind, the migration experiences of the Prague group must have been associated with an immense emotional burden. They were forced to migrate to avoid persecution, they had to depart relatively suddenly and once they had left, a return to their country of origin for 'emotional refuelling' was out of the question. Moreover, the host country was not a safe place since there was always the possibility that the Germans would invade. Constant concern for Jewish relatives and friends who had not left Germany will almost certainly have plagued the members of the Prague Group. They may also have suffered from a kind of survivor guilt. Grinberg and Grinberg speak in this context of super ego anxiety. On the other hand, the migrants in Prague were able to continue to speak and work in their own language. They were also able to continue practising their profession. The escape itself, from Berlin to Prague, was presumably relatively unproblematic. Despite the positive aspects of their migration, the members of the Prague group will certainly have experienced the emigration as extremely stressful, yet they were highly productive. We may presume that a collective manic defence played a substantial role. In this chapter, I have focused particularly on the important role of Marxism. For some of the Prague group members, psychoanalysis without Marxism had no longer seemed conceivable. The connection between psychoanalysis and Marxism can, of course, be traced back to the time of the Weimar Republic. Yet in exile, the belief in an overarching 'theory of the century', one to which one must firmly adhere, may perhaps have served a further psychodynamic function. Following the second emigration, to the US, Marxism ceased to play a significant role in the (written) discussions of the migrant psychoanalysts. While they remained in Prague, there may have been a certain group pressure to commit to Marxism despite the fact that there was no state doctrine demanding any such commitment. Furthermore, Marxism did nothing to enhance their opportunities for professional advancement. On the contrary! The pressure had come 'from the grassroots of the movement' and served no purpose beyond the group itself. Nevertheless, a non-Marxist attitude may well have been perceived as a threat to the group.

Marxist theory as understood by the group, promised to offer an all-encompassing, explanatory model. It claimed to explain overarching historical and societal processes and defined what was considered to be 'scientific' and 'progressive'. The analysts also wanted to link psychoanalysis to this theory. The idea was that the same theoretical key could be used to explain both external conditions and internal mental states. One might wonder whether there was a striving for greatness and omnipotent power inherent in such a high theoretical goal. In reality, the Prague analysts were threatened by a totalitarian regime that for them could lead not simply to repression, but to annihilation. Their situation as émigrés also confronted them with internal and external challenges. In the face of these threats and challenges, the unification of the theories of psychoanalysis and Marxism may have released an unconscious fantasy of being part of a historical force that would prevail and bring forth a better society. This would have allowed them to feel connected to a powerful and protective force. This unconscious fantasy might thus have functioned as a psychodynamic defence against painful feelings of powerlessness and exclusion. This defence mechanism might conceivably have served to protect their egos and their capacity to function. A mourning process in this situation might not have been possible or even helpful.

These thoughts are not an attempt to diagnose the emotional state, or the psychodynamics of the émigré analysts. These considerations are hypothetical. In addition, it is certainly not possible to explain the meaning that Marxism had for the group or their critique of the theory of the death instinct merely on psychodynamic grounds associated with the pressures exerted by the circumstances of their exile. Nevertheless, I believe it is quite possible – and an idea worth further consideration – that the theoretical construct of Freudo-Marxism, in combination with a strong emotional attachment to it, provided them with a necessary unconscious psychodynamic defence that helped them to deal with the emotional threats to which they were subjected. Aspects of this psychic defence are certain forms of manic defence and unconscious omnipotent fantasy. Their rejection of the concept of the death instinct took on a prominent role in their Freudo-Marxism and was emotionally highly loaded. It seems very likely to me that this rejection also had ego-protective and important psychic defence functions under these particular circumstances. I would not consider this a pathologic form of psychic defence, although it is certainly located in the realm of manic defence and unconscious omnipotent fantasy. It may nonetheless have been a quite healthy mechanism that enabled the Prague Group to function on a high level and to survive.

Notes

1. Translated by Daniel Fisher, Berlin, Kristin White, Berlin, Deirdre Winter, Berlin.
2. In German: 'Gesetz zur Wiederherstellung des Berufsbeamtentums'.
3. By that time there were already important psychoanalytic societies in various Eastern European countries. The Hungarian Psychoanalytic Society in Budapest was founded in 1913. Its members included Sándor Ferenczi, Melanie Klein, Sándor Radó and Géza Róheim. In Russia, a psychoanalytical society was founded in 1911, with a psychoanalytic outpatient clinic set up in 1917. Its members included Sabina Spielrein, Vera Schmidt and Nicolai Ossipow. Some of Freud's writings, such as the Introductory Lectures on Psychoanalysis, had already been translated into Japanese, Chinese and Hebrew before they were available in Czech in 1936 (Mühlleitner, 2008).
4. Edith Jacobson also lived in Prague for a brief period. After being arrested in 1935 as a member of the resistance group 'Neu Beginnen' (New Beginnings) and sentenced to imprisonment, she was granted parole in Berlin for health reasons and

with Fenichel's help was able to flee to Prague. She later became one of the most influential psychoanalysts of the New York Psychoanalytic Society.

5. For more details on the *Rundbriefe,* see below.
6. IPA: Internationale Psychoanalytische Vereinigung (International Psychoanalytic Association).
7. Original quote in German: 'Unter Frau Deri's Leitung wird in Prag offenbar sehr gute Arbeit geleistet. Die junge Gruppe hat zwar noch nichts publiziert, aber wir kennen ja ihre (Annie Reich, Steff Bornstein) früheren Arbeiten und Ansichten. Für die Entwicklung innerhalb der I.P.V. kann also die Aufnahme dieser Gruppe unter Umständen von ausschlaggebender Bedeutung werden. [Es] wäre ... sehr wünschenswert, daß Frau Deri sofort in Wien Mitglied würde, damit sie zum Kongress die Aufnahme der Gruppe in der I.P.V. beantragen kann.'
8. DPG: Deutsche Psychoanalytische Gesellschaft [German Psychoanalytic Society].
9. Freudo-Marxist is a translation of the German term *Freudo-Marxisten*, representatives of *Freudomarxismus*. This is an umbrella term for various theories that attempt to integrate Marxism and psychoanalysis. Important assumptions of these theories are that psychoanalysis is inherently critical of (bourgeois) society, that capitalist society and its suppression of the individual are the origin of neurosis, and that sexual and emotional freedom should be part and parcel of a revolutionary movement. Freudo-Marxism was also influential in the social movements involved in the protests that took place in Europe and the US in 1968.
10. I am putting the terms 'materialism' and 'natural science' in quotation marks here because they refer to specific and complex understandings of these terms about which there is an ongoing discussion among Marxists still today. Space does not permit a more detailed description of the use of these terms in Freudo-Marxist theories.
11. 'Die Berliner Kollegen zerstreuten sich über die ganze Welt. Wir sehnten uns nach einander und hatten gleichzeitig, – berechtigterweise – den Eindruck, daß eine Einflussnahme auf die vom Faschismus auch innerlich bedrohte psychoanalytische Bewegung nötiger war als je' (Reichmeyer and Mühlleitner, 1998, p. 16).
12. 'Seit der Todestrieblehre ist eine immer stärker werdenden Abweichung von den revolutionären empirischen Funden der Psychoanalyse fühlbar. Die ursprünglich Formel: Neurosen entstehen aus dem Zusammenprall der kindlichen Triebhaftigkeit mit den hemmenden Mächten der Gesellschaft, ist verlassen worden, an ihre Stelle treten Theorien über das Strafbedürfnis, über die Schwäche des kindlichen Ichs u. dgl. m. Die Oppositionsgruppe will die naturwissenschaftlichen Psychoanalyse, die von empirischen Beobachtungen ausgeht und die in der Libidotheorie ihren klaren Ausdruck findet, vor metaphysischen Abweichungen schützen und sie weiter konsequent ausbauen' (Reichmay and Mühlleitner, 1998, p. 86).
13. 'Ferner findet die Oppositionsgruppe, daß die Psychoanalyse ihre kulturkritische und kulturkämpferische Angabe nicht mehr erfüllt. Jene kühnen und klaren Sätze, die etwas in Freuds Aufsatz *die kulturelle Sexualmoral und die moderne Nervosität* zu finden sind und die implizit ein ganzes Programm der von der Analyse ausgehende Kulturkritik enthalten, sind vergessen' (Reichmayr and Mühlleitner, 1998, pp. 86–7).
14. 'Sie beschraenken sich zu sehr auf Kritik und geben zu wenig postives. Mir scheint, dass die wichtigste Aufgabe zunaechst darin besteht, jenen Leuten in der IPV, die nicht völlig verbloedet sind, jenes systematische Verdraengung der Realitaet, jene imbezile Verwechselung des Weltgeschens mit Behandlungsstunden bewusst zu machen, die die meisten Analytiker treiben. Dabei müssen wir nicht gleich die Realitaet marxistisch interpretieren.'

15. 'Wir sind alle davon überzeugt, in der Psychoanalyse Freuds den Keim der zukünftigen dialektisch-materialistischen Psychologie zu erkennen, und dass deshalb Pflege und Ausbau dieser Wissenschaft dringend nottun. Glaubten wir das nicht, so wären wir nicht Psychoanalytiker von Beruf. Wir sind auch weiterhin davon überzeugt, dass Pflege und Ausbau bei den Widerständen, auf die die Psychoanalyse aus bekannten Gründen stösst, am besten durch Arbeitsgemeinschaften geschieht, die ungestört von äusseren Widerständen positive Arbeit zu leisten suchen' (Reichmayr and Mühlleitner, 1998, p. 35).
16. 'Der Trieb ist derjenige Begriff, der uns jene biologischen Bedürfnisse wiederspiegelt und deshalb die unentbehrliche Brücke von unserer Wissenschaft zur Biologie darstellt. ... Einer solchen Triebdefinition will sich ein Todestrieb nicht fügen'.
17. Original: 'Ich bin dagegen, aus der Bekenntnisfrage nach dem Todestrieb allein das entscheidenen Shibboleth zu machen'.
18. Original: *Vorwort zur deutschen Ausgabe.*
19. Original: *Melanie Klein. Gesammelte Schriften.*
20. '... eine Rezeption der Theorien Melanie Kleins, die zu einer differenzierten Erforschung des destruktiven Narzissmus, der psychotischen Ängste und omnipotenten Abwehrmechanismen hätte führen können, (war [I.K.] in dieser Zeit – wenigsten in Deutschand – undenkbar' (Cycon, 1995, p. XIII).

References

Akhtar, S. (1999). *Immigration and Identity: Turmoil, Treatment, and Transformation.* Lanham, MD: Jason Aronson.

Akhtar, S. (2010). *Immigration and Acculturation: Mourning, Adaptation, and the Next Generation.* Lanham, MD: Jason Aronson.

Anastas, B. (2005). *Am Fuß des Gebirges.* Vienna: Jung und Jung.

Becher, P. (ed.) (1989). *Drehscheibe Prag. Deutsche Emigranten 1933–1939. Ausstellungskatalog.* Munich: Adalbert Stifter Verein.

Becher, P., and Heumos, P. (eds) (1992). *Drehscheiber Prag: Zur Deutsche Emigration in der Tschechoslowakei (1933–1939).* Munich: Oldenbourg Verlag.

Beltsiou, J. (ed.) (2016). *Immigration in Psychoanalysis. Locating Ourselves.* Abingdon and New York: Routledge.

Cycon, R. (ed.) (1995). *Melanie Klein. Gesammelte Schriften, Vol. 1.* Stuttgart-Bad Cannstatt: Fromman-Holzboog.

Fischer, E. (1992). Czechoslovakia. In P. Kuttner (ed.), *Psychoanalysis International Vol. I: A Guide to Psychoanalysis Throughout the World.* Stuttgart-Bad Cannstatt: Frommann-Holzboog.

Freud, S. (1900). The Interpretation of Dreams. *Standard Edition, Vol. IV* (pp. ix–627). London: Hogarth Press.

Grinberg, L., and Grinberg, R. (1989). *Psychoanalytic Perspectives on Migration and Exile,* New Haven, CT: Yale University Press.

Jacoby, R. (1985). *Die Verdrängung der Psychoanalyse oder der Triumph des Konformismus.* Frankfurt am Main: Fischer. Originally published as *The Repression of Psychoanalysis: Otto Fenichel and the Political Freudians.* New York: Basic Books Inc., 1983.

Krohn, C. (ed.) (2002). *Metropolen des Exils. Exil Forschung. Ein Internationales Jahrbuch. Vol. 20.* Munich: Edition Text und Kritik.

Kuriloff, E.A. (2014). *Contemporary Psychoanalysis and the Legacy of the Third Reich: History, Memory, Tradition*. New York: Routledge.

Lockot, R. (2003). *Erinnern und Durcharbeiten*. Gießen: Psychosozial Verlag.

Lockot, R. (1994). *Die Reinigung der Psychoanalyse*. Gießen: Psychosozial Verlag.

Ludwig-Körner, C. (1998). *Wiederentdeckt – Psychoanalytikerinnen in Berlin*. Gießen: Psychosozial Verlag.

Marx, K. (1859/2010) A Contribution to the Critique of Political Economy. In Terrell Karver (ed.), *Karl Marx: Later Political Writings*. Cambridge: Cambridge University Press.

Mühlleitner, E. (1992). *Biographisches Lexikon der Psychoanalyse*. Tübingen: edition diskord.

Mühlleitner, E. (2000). Steff Bornstein, Otto Fenichel und die psychoanalytisch-pädagogische Ausbildung der Psychoanalytischen Arbeitsgemeinschaft v. C.S.R. (1933–1939). In *Luzifer-Amor 13*(25), S. 64–77. Frankfurt am Main: Brandes & Apsel.

Mühlleitner, E. (2008). *Ich – Fenichel. Das Leben eines Psychoanalytikers im 20. Jahrhundert*. Vienna: Paul Zsolnay Verlag.

Müller, T. (2000). *Von Charlottenburg zum Central Park West. Henry Lowenfeld und die Psychoanalyse in Berlin, Prag und New York*. Frankfurt am Main.: Edition Déjà vu.

Reichmayr, J., and Mühlleitner, E. (eds) (1998). *Otto Fenichel 119 Rundbriefe, Vol. 1*, Europa (1934–1938). Frankfurt am Main and Basel: Stroemfeld.

Reinerová, L. (2006). *Es begann in der Melantrichgasse*. Berlin: Aufbau-Verlag.

Röder, W. (1992). Drehscheibe – Kampfposten – Fluchtstation. Deutsche Emigranten in der Tschechoslowakei. In Becher, P., and Heumos, P. (eds), (1992), *Drehscheiber Prag: Zur Deutsche Emigration in der Tschechoslowakei (1933–1939)*. Munich: Oldenbourg Verlag.

Schneider, C. (1999). Der Mann, der Freud und Marx zusammenbringen wollte. *Baseler Zeitung*, 29. May 1999.

Šebek, M. (2013). Psychoanalyse in Tschechien. Äußere Realität und Verdrängung. *Psyche, Zeitschrift für Psychoanalyse und ihre Anwendung*. Jahrgang 67 Heft 3 S.238–250. Frankfurt a.M.: Klett Cotta.

Weil, J. (1995). *Leben mit dem Stern*. Reinbeck bei Hamburg: Rowohlt Taschenbuchverlag.

Select bibliography

Akhtar, S. (1999). *Immigration and Identity: Turmoil, Treatment, and Transformation*. Northvale, NJ: Jason Aronson.

Amati-Mehler, J., Argentieri, S., and Canestri, J. (1993). *Babel of the Unconscious: Mother Tongue and Foreign Languages in the Psychoanalytic Dimension*, trans. J. Whitelaw Cucco. Madison, CT: International Universities Press.

Arendt, H. (1943). We Refugees. *Menorah Journal*.

Arendt, H. (2018). *Wir Flüchtlinge – mit einem Essay von Thomas Meyer*. Stuttgart: Reclam.

Beltsiou, J. (ed.) (2016). *Immigration in Psychoanalysis: Locating Ourselves*. Abingdon and New York: Routledge.

Blos, P. (1963). *On Adolescence – A Psychoanalytic Interpretation*. New York: Free Press of Glencoe.

Cogoy, R. (2001). Fremdheit und interkulturelle Kommunikation in der Psychotherapie. *Psyche – Zeitschrift für Psychoanalyse und ihre Anwendungen*, *55*(4), 339–57.

Davids, M.F. (2011). *Internal Racism: A Psychoanalytic Approach to Race and Difference*. Basingstoke: Palgrave Macmillan.

Erpenbeck, J. (2017). *Go, Went, Gone*, trans. Susan Bernofsky. London: Granta.

Fonagy, P., Gergely, G., Jurist, E.L., and Target, M. (2002). *Affect Regulation, Mentalization and the Development of the Self*. New York: Other Press.

Freud, S. (1900). The Interpretation of Dreams. *Standard Edition, Vol. IV*. London: Hogarth Press.

Freud, S. (1917). Mourning and Melancholia. *Standard Edition, Vol. XIV* (pp. 237–58). London: Hogarth Press.

Freud, S. (1927). Fetishism. *Standard Edition, Vol. XXI* (pp. 147–57). London: Hogarth Press.

Garza-Guerrero, A.C. (1974). Culture shock: its mourning and the vicissitudes of identity. *Journal of the American Psychoanalytic Association*, *22*(2), 408–29.

Gay, P. ([1998]2006). *Freud: A Life for Our Time*. London: W.W. Norton & Co.

Grinberg, L. and Grinberg, R. (1984). *Psychoanalytic Perspectives on Migration and Exile*. New Haven and London: Yale University Press.

Kareem, J. (1992). The Nafsiyat Intercultural Therapy Centre: Ideas and Experience in Intercultural Therapy. In J. Kareem and R. Littlewood (eds), *Intercultural Therapy: Themes, Interpretations and Practice*. Oxford: Blackwell Scientific Publications.

King, P. and Steiner, R. (eds.) (1991). The Freud-Klein Controversies 1941–45. *New Library of Psychoanalysis*, *11*: 1–942. London and New York: Tavistock/Routledge.

Klein, M. (1932). The Psycho-Analysis of Children. *The International Psycho-Analytical Library*, *22*: 1–379. London: The Hogarth Press.

Kogan, I. (1995). *The Cry of Mute Children: A Psychoanalytic Perspective of the Second Generation of the Holocaust*. London and New York: Free Association Books.

Kogan, I. (2007). *The Struggle against Mourning*. Plymouth: Jason Aronson and Lanham, MD: Rowman and Littlefield.

Kuriloff, E.A. (2014). *Contemporary Psychoanalysis and the Legacy of the Third Reich: History, Memory, Tradition*. New York: Routledge.

Leary, K. (2000). Racial enactments in dynamic treatment. *Psychoanalytic Dialogues*, *10*(4), 639–53.

Meisel, P. and Kendrick, W. (eds), (1985) *Bloomsbury/Freud: The Letters of James and Alix Strachey, 1924–1925*. New York: Basic Books

Parin, P. (1988). The Ego and the Mechanisms of Adaptation. In Boyer, B. and Grolnik, S.A. (eds), *The Psychoanalytic Study of Society, Vol. 12*. Hillsdale, NJ: The Analytic Press.

Reichmayr, J. and Mühlleitner, E. (eds) (1988). *Otto Fenichel 119 Rundbriefe, Vol. 1, Europa (1934–1938)*. Frankfurt am Main and Basel: Stroemfeld.

Reichmayr, J. and Mühlleitner, E. (eds) (1988a). *Otto Fenichel 119 Rundbriefe, Vol. 2, Amerika (1938–1945)*. Frankfurt am Main and Basel: Stroemfeld.

Rustin, M. (2013). Finding Out Where and Who One Is: The Special Complexity of Migration for Adolescents. In Varchevker, A. and McGinley, E. (eds), *Enduring Migration through the Life Cycle*. London: Karnac.

Segal, H. (1991). *Dream, Phantasy and Art*. London: Routledge.

Steiner, J. (1993). *Psychic Retreats*. London: Routledge.

Volkan, V.D. (1993). Immigrants and refugees: A psychoanalytic perspective. *Mind and Human Interaction*, *4*, 63–9.

Waddell, M. ([1998]2019). *Inside Lives: Psychoanalysis and the Growth of the Personality*. London: Routledge.

Waddell, M. (2018). *On Adolescence: Inside Stories*. Tavistock Clinic Series. London: Routledge.

Index

Note: page numbers followed by n refer to notes.